HEALTH-SEEKERS IN THE SOUTHWEST, 1817–1900

Health-Seekers in the Southwest, 1817-1900

by Billy M. Jones

UNIVERSITY OF OKLAHOMA PRESS : NORMAN

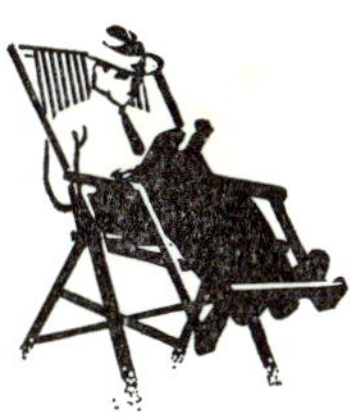

BY BILLY M. JONES

The Search for Maturity: The Saga of Texas, 1875–1900 (Austin, 1965)
Health-Seekers in the Southwest, 1817–1900 (Norman, 1967)

LIBRARY OF CONGRESS CATALOG CARD NUMBER: 67–15572

 Composed and printed at Norman, Oklahoma, U.S.A., by the University of Oklahoma Press. First edition.

For the Joneses I try to keep up with

DORIS, JEFF, WOODY,
RUSTY, AND SCOTTY

Preface

TRADITION has preserved and legend has dramatized the more spectacular reasons for westward immigration; indeed, historians, following the oft-quoted Frederick Jackson Turner, have thoroughly analyzed the motives of virtually every group of pioneers who settled and developed the West. Overlooked, however—in fact, utterly ignored as an important factor in population movements during the nineteenth century—was the relentless quest for health by hundreds of thousands of disease-ridden Americans. This neglected but persistent characteristic of the century nevertheless is highly significant to the study of American frontier history.

The presence of such large numbers of health-seekers in the frontier movement indicates that nineteenth-century Americans faced serious health problems, which medical science proved incapable of solving. The failure of formal medicine to provide adequate relief even for simple diseases forced laymen and doctors alike to place great reliance upon changes of residence or therapeutic travel as the surest means of dissipating a persistent illness or of avoiding the contaminations of an infectious location.

A pragmatic, century-long search for a health-restoring and disease-free area led inevitably to the early discovery and subsequent development of what many pioneers referred to as nature's sanatorium, the elevated, moistureless, sun-drenched plains and mountains health frontier in the lower Southwest. Early invalid residents of the region migrated principally from the Mississippi Basin, an incredibly rich series of river valleys which unfortunately were found to be extremely unhealthy. The bulk of later health travelers were the pitiable tubercular victims of overcrowded slum areas and sweat-shop factories in the newly industrialized East. Together, these groups constituted some 20 to 25 per cent of total immigration to the Southwest during the nineteenth century, and both contributed to the development of most of the states and territories in that region.

Twentieth-century Americans continue to acknowledge, and to take advantage of, the healthful climate of the Southwest, but they are, for the most part, completely unaware of the "golden era of invalidism" and its influence upon the institutional and cultural history of the West. Thus, this book seeks to trace the growth of the western health frontier, to analyze the importance and impact of health-seeking in the development of the Southwest, and to explain the probable reasons why the search for health has been consistently ignored in all historical analyses of the period.

Now obsolescent terminology is frequently used in the text in order to preserve the flavor of nineteenth-century medical language. The most prominent of these are ague (malaria), bilious fever (dysentery), phthisis (consumption or tuberculosis), miasmata (fogs, vapors, and effluvia arising from swamps or from the decomposition of vegetable and animal matter), and climatology (the study of climate and its alterative effects upon specific diseases, particularly tuberculosis).

During the course of my labors, I have incurred many debts for assistance. To Professor Seymour V. Connor goes a special word of thanks for giving unselfishly of his limited time and extensive talents during the preparation of this work, as well as to the staff of the Southwest Collection, research center at Texas Technological College, which he formerly headed. Additionally, I am grateful to Professors Lowell L. Blaisdell, J. William Davis, Lawrence L. Graves, W. Curry Holden, W. Eugene Hollon, David M. Vigness, and Ernest Wallace for reading the manuscript and offering criticisms as well as encouragement. I must express appreciation also to Mrs. Shirley Reese and Mrs. Virginia Scott for typing the manuscript at various stages, and to Ray Janeway of Texas Technological College, a librarian of the first rank, for the professional and sympathetic assistance he always gives to those who are in search of elusive research materials.

For invaluable assistance in locating, and to their respective institutions for permission to reproduce, appropriate photographs, a final note of appreciation is expressed to Mrs. Alys Freeze, Head, Western History Department of the Denver Public Library; to Mrs. Barbara Kelso, Acting Librarian, University of Texas, Medical Branch, Galveston, Texas; and to Mr. Bert Fireman, Executive Vice-President of the Arizona Historical Foundation.

BILLY M. JONES

San Angelo, Texas
January 26, 1967

Contents

Illustrations

HEALTH-SEEKERS IN THE SOUTHWEST, 1817–1900

I. *The Valley of Frustration*

THE GREATEST OBSTRUCTION to the settlement of the trans-Appalachian frontier was not the prodigious vegetation to be cleared nor the limitless timber lands to be razed nor even the hostile Indians to be subdued; instead, it was the creeping, silent menace of poor health and disease. Bravery and hard work quickly removed most obstacles, but there were no weapons men could use against the plethora of deadly infections which raged from one end of the Mississippi Valley to the other, "seeking whom they [might] destroy."[1]

So evident was this danger that one author wrote: "The entire colonization of the Mississippi Valley, from Pittsburg[h] to Middle Kansas, a width of 1,000 miles, has been carried on with the almost universal accompaniment of fevers."[2] Indeed, in attempting to determine the geographical limits of autumnal fevers (malaria and dysentery), one of the most reliable medical observers in the interior valley found that no part of the greater Mississippi Basin was exempt from the ravages of the fevers:

1 William Newnham Blaney, "An Excursion Through the U.S. and Canada 1822–23," as abridged in Harlow Lindley (ed.), *Indiana as Seen by Early Travelers* (hereafter referred to as *Indiana Travelers*), 285. By 1800, disease was regarded as a far greater menace to the settlement of Illinois than the Indians. Isaac D. Rawlings, *The Rise and Fall of Disease in Illinois*, I, 29.

2 William G. Ritch, *New Mexico, Historical and Industrial*, 67.

> . . . in every other direction than the south, this endemic has its geographical limits. To the east, its barrier is the Appalachian Mountains, into the very gorges of which, however, its ascends by the valleys which penetrate their flanks. . . . To the southwest the Cordilleras of Mexico, and the Southern Rocky Mountains, constitute its boundaries; while in the lower latitudes, it ceases on the great plains of our western desert, long before we reach those Mountains.[3]

Thus the Mississippi Valley was, in a pioneer colloquialism, well below the fever line.

From the earliest period of immigration, health—or the lack of it—was a prominent pioneer concern; sickness was the most commonly used word for caution and health the yardstick by which happiness was measured. Fevers were so prevalent that nearly every Valley state "cherished legends of remote villages where church bells rang every day at noon to remind people to take their quinine." And as the Mississippi Valley's reputation for unhealthfulness became both widespread and justified, it became an important factor to be weighed against the powerful appeals of "freedom and fortune" offered by the new lands. Little wonder that cautious immigrants subjected almost every square mile of the greater Mississippi Valley to the closest scrutiny, always testing and weighing in their minds the salubrity of each region.[4]

From both general observations and personal experiences, immigrants came to respect an overriding truth about western lands, one which made the selection of a healthful location a frustrating experience: nature seemed everywhere to be in a state of disequilibrium. In regions where conditions were found to be most favorable to health, there was a definite lack of adequate farm-

[3] Daniel Drake, M.D., *A Systematic Treatise . . . on the Principal Diseases of the Interior Valley of North America*, 704.

[4] Albert D. Richardson, *Beyond the Mississippi: From the Great River to the Great Ocean*, 132; R. Carlyle Buley, *The Old Northwest: Pioneer Period: 1815–1840*, I, 240.

ing lands, and where deep, fertile soils were found, good health was not. At Wheeling, [West] Virginia, located on the western slope of the Allegheny Mountains, one of the older inhabitants was asked if the country was healthy. "Healthy, sir!" he replied, "that it is—healthy and poor—ten people run away where one dies in it."[5]

The poor-soil good-health truism was sharply reversed in settlements beyond the mountains. Travelers in the westerly areas were constantly shocked by the "sallow complexions, the withered features, and the fleshless, ague-racked limbs which . . . [peeped] forth . . . from the luxuriant foliage of this region of sepulchures." So pronounced was the contrast that Timothy Flint wrote in 1832: "There appears to be in the great plan of Providence a scale in which the advantages and disadvantages of human condition are balanced. Where the lands are extremely fertile, it seems appended to them . . . that they are generally sickly."[6]

Increasing familiarity with the attributes of western lands developed an important thesis: infestation was more directly related to location than to climate, though both frequently were referred to concomitantly. But if immigrants learned pragmatically to classify certain areas as unhealthy, they were none too certain of the reasons why they did so; the causes of most diseases were among nature's best-kept secrets. The most commonly held view in the early nineteenth century was that the fogs and vapors which hovered about stagnant waters, swamps, and muddy river bottoms, and the miasmata and effluvia which arose from the decomposition of vegetable and animal matter were

[5] Charles Fenno Hoffman, *A Winter in the West,* I, 46.

[6] Edmund Flagg, *The Far West: or, a Tour Beyond the Mountains,* in Reuben Gold Thwaites (ed.), *Early Western Travels, 1748–1846* (hereafter referred to as *Early Western Travels*), XXVI, 126; Timothy Flint, *The History and Geography of the Mississippi Valley,* I, 36.

the chief causes of physical disorders.[7] Pioneers were aware, however, of the swarms of mosquitoes, blowflies, gnats, fleas, lice, ticks, worms, rats, lizards, frogs, and snakes which abounded throughout the Valley, but for the most part neither the early settler nor the medical profession recognized these pests as a principal source of disease and infection. The most frequently encountered of these infectious creatures was the mosquito, yet despite its omnipresence it was regarded only as an abominable and unavoidable nuisance.[8]

From the fertile river bottoms and rolling prairies to the more marginal lands in timbered and mountainous regions, the search for a healthy location continued for at least half of the nineteenth century. By then the evidence of the "blight on the Valley" was well known. Scarcely any type of terrain or physical category had escaped the pioneers' indictment, and even the few places not branded as unhealthy often were described only as relatively, not absolutely, free from disease.

River valleys especially bore a label of gross insalubrity after experience revealed that even the best navigable waters and the healthiest locations were "incompatible, and seldom admitting of immediate proximity to one another." Most feared were those areas near the rivers where stagnant waters and creeping bayous were entrapped, and prospective settlers were constantly warned not to construct residences near them. Additionally, river bottoms and alluvial deposits adjacent to the banks proved to be

[7] See for example: Morris Birkbeck, "Notes on a Journey . . . to the Territory of Illinois (1818)," in Lindley's *Indiana Travelers,* 176; Edwin James, *Account of an Expedition to the Rocky Mountains,* in Thwaites' *Early Western Travels,* XVII, 129; François Marie Perrin du Lac, *Travel Through the Two Louisianas,* 7; John Regan, *The Emigrant's Guide to the Western States of America,* 394; John W. Monnette, *History of the Discovery and Settlement of the Valley of the Mississippi,* I, 486.

[8] Amos Andrew Parker, *Trip to the West and Texas,* 109. For an impassioned condemnation of "the greatest torment [the mosquito] that was ever sent to afflict man for his iniquities," see Jabez Wiggins Heustis, *Physical Observations . . . on the Topography and Diseases of Louisiana,* 41–42.

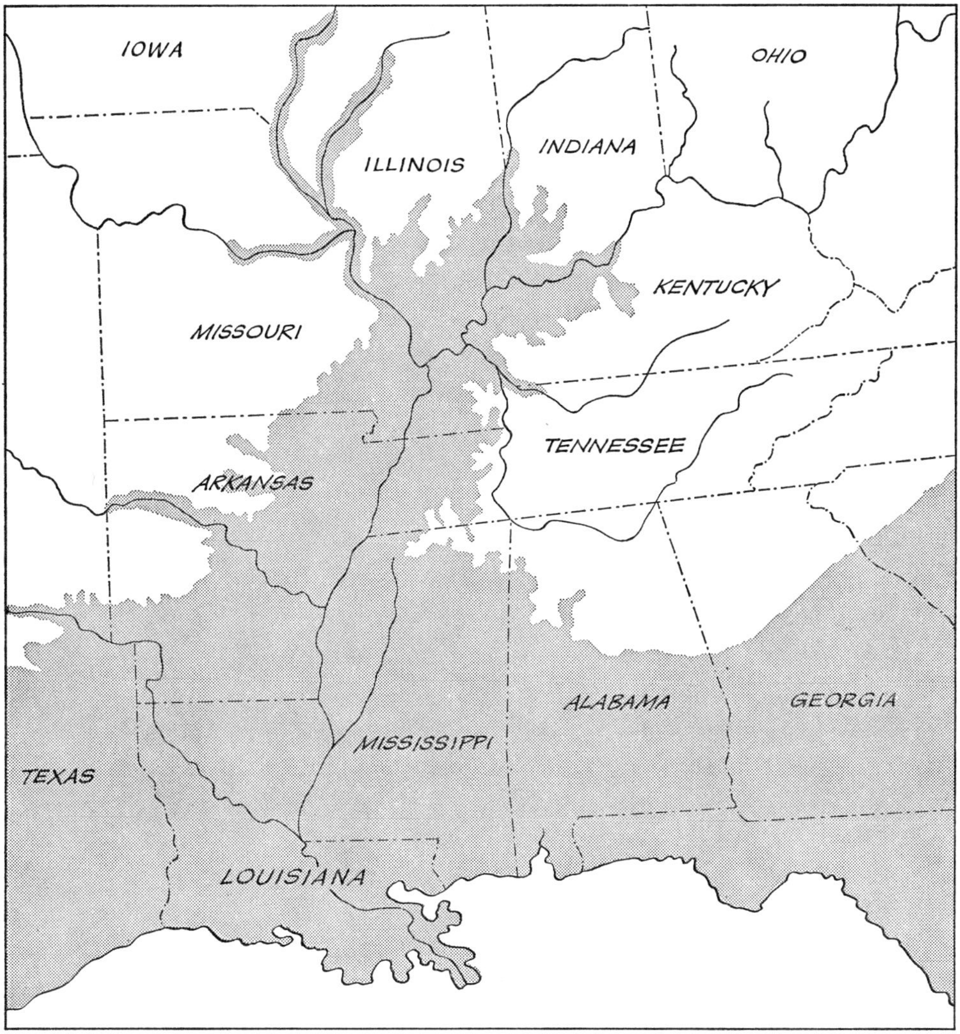

THE GREATER MISSISSIPPI BASIN

dangerous sites, though their excellent fertility was a constant, and often fatal, attraction to hopeful farmers.[9]

Descriptions by contemporary travelers of their experiences on the principal waterways should have discouraged all but the most courageous emigrants, yet one writer remarked that other types of terrain would "never draw inhabitants . . . while a foot of cane brake or river bottom remains to be settled." The Mississippi, described by Charles Dickens as "an enormous ditch, sometimes two or three miles wide, running liquid mud" and a "breeding-place of fever, ague, and death," was always settled somewhat incautiously. Charles Murray, after landing some twenty times along the banks of the Missouri, was unable to find "a single family where the fever and ague had not chased the natural colour from their cheeks." He found it hard to believe that "they would outlive another season." One traveler along the Ohio River saw only dirty, sickly children; another found the Wabash Valley filled with settlers whose countenances "bespeak how often they have been attacked" by diseases; still another found the Arkansas, whose sides were covered with sleeping lakes and stagnant bayous, "too often . . . [visited] of bilious and remittent fevers" to admit a large population.[10]

River towns such as Chillicothe (Illinois), Cincinnati, Louisville, Terre Haute, St. Louis, Memphis, Natchez, and New Orleans offered little protection from the general insalubrity of the

[9] James Flint, *Letters from America,* in Thwaites' *Early Western Travels,* IX, 189; T. Flint, *History . . . of the Mississippi Valley,* I, 36; David Thomas, "Travels Through the Western Country in the Summer of 1816," in Lindley's *Indiana Travelers,* 121.

[10] Fortescue Cuming, *Sketches of a Tour to the Western Country,* in Thwaites' *Early Western Travels,* IV, 351; Charles Dickens, *American Notes,* 249; Charles Augustus Murray, *Travels in North America,* II, 84; John Woods, *Two Years' Residence . . . in the Illinois Country, United States,* in Thwaites' *Early Western Travels,* X, 247; Blaney, "An Excursion Through the U.S. and Canada 1822–23," in Lindley's *Indiana Travelers,* 285; T. Flint, *History . . . of the Mississippi Valley,* I, 281. Another of the tributaries of the Mississippi bears the name Yazoo, which, in the language of the Choctaw Indian, means "River of Death." Frank E. Smith, *The Yazoo River, xvi.*

waterways on which they were located, all of them being described at one time or another as exceedingly unhealthy. Although these towns attained early prominence, others were less fortunate. In fact, some townsites eventually were abandoned because of their unhealthful locations, and others declined slowly in population for the same reason.[11]

Prairie lands, no less than river valleys, were found to be disease infested. Often low-lying and wet, almost denuded of trees, and invariably covered with a variety of grasses and weeds, these champaigns extended over parts of Ohio, Kentucky, and Tennessee, large sections of Indiana, Illinois, and Missouri, even greater portions of Mississippi and Arkansas, and nearly all of Louisiana. Too often such lands did not have sufficient slope to carry off rain water and thus were ready breeding places for all types of insects and pests. Their waters were discharged, especially during the hot summer months, through evaporation, a process which accentuated the swampish vapors and effluvia so feared by settlers. The fact that fevers and ague were constant companions to those who dared to settle on these prairie lands gave rise to a reputation for unhealthiness "too well founded to admit of refutation." Although large portions of prairie lands remained for a time " almost entirely destitute of inhabitants," the ease with which settlements could be formed on them attracted a steady stream of farmers and stock raisers.[12]

Most celebrated of the champaign regions were the Mississippi bottoms, located in the low area in southern Illinois toward which the Ohio, Tennessee, Wabash, Kaskaskia, Missouri, and Mississippi rivers drain. The union of these rivers during violent floods

[11] Woods, *Two Years' Residence, Early Western Travels,* X, 266n., 326, 327n., 328; Blaney, "An Excursion Through the U.S. and Canada 1822–23," *Indiana Travelers,* 281.

[12] T. Flint, *History . . . of the Mississippi Valley,* I, 318; E. James, *Account of an Expedition, Early Western Travels,* XVII, 111; Thomas Scattergood Teas, "Journal of a Tour to Fort Wayne . . . in the Year 1821," in Lindley's *Indiana Travelers,* 247.

has flushed out a large inland lake bed. The gift of their floods is rich alluvial topsoil, the curse poor drainage. All pioneers who braved the incongruities of this region fled in frustration; not even the Trappists, most persevering and ascetic of all Roman Catholic monks, were able to endure the unhealthfulness of the bottoms.[13]

Settlers who inadvertently found a healthful location in timbered regions did so not so much from woodland surroundings as from elevation. They were often disappointed to find in the lower areas an atmosphere which was "close and unelastic" and only slightly more advantageous than that of the surrounding prairies. Yet in the higher sections, better health had to be balanced against an old nemesis—poorer soils. The most favorable of such locations for both material and physical well-being was found to be at the edge of the prairies, with open land for agricultural pursuits and woods as a home site. Even then, happiness was found to be precariously balanced between profit and peril.[14]

Thus it developed that the best health was always associated with a degree of elevation and especially with the mountainous regions of western Pennsylvania, Kentucky, Tennessee, and Arkansas. Additionally, the high, rolling country located at some distance from the rivers was well regarded. Usually well-drained, often supplied with clear spring water, and frequently possessed of good soil, these higher lands rapidly acquired greater numbers of people and became centers of thriving communities. Elevation, however, had its limitations, as did all types of terrain, for a partial elevation of ground in an unhealthy district proved at

[13] T. Flint, *History . . . of the Mississippi Valley,* I, 128; Flagg, *The Far West, Early Western Travels,* XXVI, 193–94. The unhealthfulness of the Mississippi Bottoms was the major reason why early pioneers referred to Illinois as a "graveyard." John Reynolds, *Reynolds' History of Illinois,* 44.

[14] T. Flint, *History . . . of the Mississippi Valley,* I, 40 ff.; Richard Flower, *Letters from Lexington and the Illinois,* in Thwaites' *Early Western Travels,* X, 129; Cuming, *Sketches of a Tour, ibid.,* IV, 351; J. Flint, *Letters from America, ibid.,* IX, 130.

times to be more pernicious than the lower ground around it. The cause of this dilemma was fixed upon contaminated air transported by winds from the surrounding area, air which had not become "sufficiently diluted with the atmosphere" of the higher region. The remedy was to withdraw a greater distance from the source of contagion, preferably into the higher country.[15] Thus, a change of location eventually came to be recognized as the best prescription in remedial as well as preventive medicine.

Much of the apparent universality of sickly conditions in the greater Mississippi Valley can be explained by the physical makeup of the Valley itself. In reality, the Mississippi Basin is a vast drainage system, capable of carrying off the combined waters of the rivers flowing west and east from the Appalachian and Rocky Mountains, respectively. As such the Basin has been subjected for centuries to the combined floodwater turbulence of many great rivers, an action which has created a vast mid-continent trough, no part of which is higher than four hundred feet above sea level. The Basin, of which the Mississippi River is but a part, has become in effect an immense, swampy river bottom without definite shore lines.[16]

Such a great, low-lying sluice could be expected to impose its conditions upon surrounding and supporting areas, and it did. The Valley became, among other things, the largest carrier of diseases in America during the nineteenth century; epidemics which began in one area were rapidly transmitted throughout the length of the entire Valley.[17] Endemics were shared in common by all regions adjacent to the mighty Mississippi.

[15] Isaac Reed, "The Christian Traveler, 1828," in Lindley's *Indiana Travelers*, 499; E. James, *Account of an Expedition, Early Western Travels*, XVII, 108; W. Bullock, *A Sketch of a Journey Through the Western States*, *ibid.*, XIX, 131; J. Flint, *Letters from America*, *ibid.*, IX, 184, 189.

[16] For an early and excellent study of the mutualities of the rivers of the Mississippi Valley, see James K. Hosmer, *A Short History of the Mississippi Valley*, Chapter I.

[17] E. James, *Account of an Expedition, Early Western Travels*, XVII, 119; Bullock, *A Sketch of a Journey*, *ibid.*, XIX, 131.

Thus diseases in the Valley were seldom discerning, striking whoever was available whenever conditions were favorable. Strangers, however, were much more susceptible than natives to the ravages of the new country. All newcomers, regardless of the time of year, faced a seasoning period during which they were subjected to a feverish conditioning to their new surroundings. Further, older inhabitants as well as new settlers had to endure an annual "sickly season"—a period lasting usually from July to October—during which fevers and ague raged almost unchecked. Affliction in one season gave no assurance of immunization during the next, although there was a gradual lessening of the severity of subsequent attacks until a person became fully acclimated or wasted away and died.[18]

Theories concerning the length of the acclimation period ranged from a few years to almost a lifetime. At New Orleans it was held that "nine years must elapse before one becomes entirely used to the effects of the swamps which surround the town." On the other hand, an old settler in the Wabash Valley once declared that he had "suffered from [fevers] every season for twenty-seven years."[19]

Seasoned natives were easy to distinguish from the newer settlers, for their emaciated frames and "meagre, tawney viasages" contrasted sharply with the plump bodies and ruddy complexions of the uninitiated. One "conditioned" resident upon whom the fevers had done their appointed work was once described as "shuck up and doubled up, too . . . that perfect wreck, a thoroughly acclimated man." He was, in local terminology, "yaller behind the gills; his face was of a pale orange tint, his cheeks

[18] Amos Stoddard, *Sketches, Historical and Descriptive, of Louisiana,* 170; Cuming, *Sketches of a Tour, Early Western Travels,* IV, 349; Alex Mackay, *The Western World: Travels in the U.S. in 1846–47,* 302.

[19] Emmanuel H. D. Domenech, *Seven Years' Residence in the Great Deserts of North America,* I, 105; Richardson, *Beyond the Mississippi,* 132.

a dirty saffron, while along the neck his skin resembled a ripe pumpkin spreckled with coffee grounds." Although he was considered the worst "shook up" settler in his area, he still had a "heap o' life left in him yet."[20]

The scourge of the Valley and the terror of the sickly months were bilious fevers and ague—the former dysenteric, the latter malarial, in nature. Referred to as autumnal fevers, these maladies appeared during the late summer and attacked a staggering proportion of Valley residents until the chilly winds of November cleared the atmosphere. Often entire families became bedridden, leaving no one well enough to care for the remaining members. Worse, the fevers seemed "to commit their greatest devastations amongst the young and the strong." Survivors frequently were "rendered unfit for labor for three or four months, and many received irreparable injury to their constitutions." The racking chills, excruciating headaches, heavy sweating, and intense body pain which accompanied the fevers so often debilitated a patient that he became an easy prey to even worse afflictions such as jaundice and dropsy. By far the most serious, and certainly the most feared, of the residual diseases was consumption or phthisis, a disease known today as tuberculosis and one for which there was then no cure.[21]

In addition to these endemic infections, the early pioneers brought with them the afflictions of the older communities of the East. Scarlet fever, diphtheria, measles, mumps, smallpox, erysipelas, pneumonia, and typhoid epidemics frequently harassed nearly every community. Skin eruptions many times worse than the itch, and milk sickness, a deadly "puking fever" con-

[20] C. F. Volney, "A View of the Soil and Climate of the United States of America (1804)," in Lindley's *Indiana Travelers,* 19; J. H. Beadle, *Western Wilds and the Men Who Redeem Them,* 26.

[21] J. Flint, *Letters from America, Early Western Travels,* IX, 288; Cuming, *Sketches of a Tour, ibid.,* IV, 349; Flagg, *The Far West,* ibid., XXVII, 96.

tracted by drinking milk from cows that fed on white snakeroot and rayless goldenrod, were encountered in many localities. This last disease always claimed its victims quickly and sometimes left its devastating marks by completely depopulating small villages.[22]

Most feared of the Valley epidemics were Asiatic cholera and yellow fever, both of which raged unchecked up and down the Valley at varying intervals during the nineteenth century. Brought to the United States via China, Russia, Europe, and Canada, the cholera staged at least two demoralizing raids upon Valley residents first in 1832 and again in 1848, the initial seige lasting two years and the second lingering sporadically for eight. The decks of river boats were swept clean of both passengers and deck hands, and cities were virtually paralyzed by the effects of this Asiatic intruder. When John Wyeth, a Valley traveler in 1832, saw more people dying in New Orleans than could be buried, he was moved to take employment as a gravedigger and for a month helped prepare huge graves, each having a capacity of three hundred bodies.[23]

Many of those who fell during the 1832 epidemic in New Orleans were victims of both cholera and yellow fever, the latter an annual plague of the Crescent City. Imported from the Caribbean seacoast and island towns, the "black vomit" reached epidemic level almost every summer, and more than one thousand deaths a year were attributed to it during the period 1825–60. Moreover, whenever New Orleans became heavily infested with yellow fever, the Mississippi Valley vibrated "for a thousand

[22] Madge E. Pickard and R. Carlyle Buley, *The Midwest Pioneer: His Ills, Cures and Doctors,* 21–22; Hoffman, *A Winter in the West,* II, 69. Nancy Hanks Lincoln, mother of Abraham Lincoln, died suddenly from milk sickness in 1818. William E. Wilson, *The Wabash,* 211.

[23] John Duffy (ed.), *The Rudolph Matas History of Medicine in Louisiana,* I, 138–40; John B. Wyeth, *Oregon; or a Short History of a Long Journey,* in Thwaites' *Early Western Travels,* XXI, 92.

miles upstream" from the effects of the disease.[24] Relief from this most fatal of all the early epidemic diseases was not to come until the twentieth century.

Persons like Wyeth, who traveled throughout the western country as observers and later wrote of their experiences, were truly stunned by the number of sick people they encountered. "I never saw," one of them wrote, "the same number of persons look so languid, emaciated and sick." Another reported seeing more sick people during a twenty-day visit to Missouri than in the whole of his preceding life in Kentucky.[25] Many writers were so moved by what they saw that they felt obligated to warn their readers of the enormity of the struggle against disease and death. "The report of a traveller," wrote David Thomas, "which may influence the emigrant, ought to embrace 'the truth and the whole truth' . . . it ought not to be concealed that at present in this country there are many sick people." Adelard Welby warned, "Let none forget that the comforts of life are more than cent per cent dearer [in the western country] than in the eastern States; and [that] health is far more likely to be preserved in the old settled country." Henry Schoolcraft, quoting a friend, wrote: "In this country [Illinois] life is at least fifty percent below par in the months of August and September," and he concluded that no army had ever suffered a greater proportion of casualties in any campaign than the inhabitants had in one of their yearly battles against disease. Wyeth admonished: "Reader! The book you hold in your hands is not written for your amusement . . . but for your instruction, particularly to warn young farmers . . .

24 Duffy, *History of Medicine in Louisiana*, I, 123–24; Estwick Evans, *A Pedestrious Tour, of Four Thousand Miles Through the Western States and Territories*, in Thwaites' *Early Western Travels*, VIII, 314; Stoddard, *Sketches . . . of Louisiana*, 170.

25 Thomas Ashe, "Travels in America Performed in 1806," in Lindley's *Indiana Travelers*, 27; J. Flint, *Letters from America, Early Western Travels*, IX, 130.

not to leave a certainty for an uncertainty."[26] Perhaps the truth in these warnings is best summed up by the "Song of the Valley," written before mid-century:

To the West! to the West! I once went, do you see
And one visit, I'm sure, was sufficient for me;
Oh, the things that I saw there, they frightened me quite
And ever since then, sirs, I've scarcely been right.

My children got sick every day, sirs, almost
And my wife took the chills, and got deaf as a post;
Oh, there's some may exalt, but for me, sirs, I'm blessed
If I haven't as much as I want of the West.[27]

Many of the itinerant scribes qualified as experts on the subject of Valley diseases, having fallen victim themselves to one of the many prevalent infections. Among those humbled by bilious fevers and ague were John Bradbury, Tilly Buttrick, Major S. H. Long, Schoolcraft, and Mrs. Frances Trollope; by yellow fever, Perrin du Lac, Benjamin Latrobe, and Wyeth; by cholera, Maximilian, prince of Wied; and by consumption, Timothy Flint. Some of them feared their afflictions would be fatal; Bradbury wrote that he did not expect to recover and Schoolcraft that he did not expect ever to pen another line in a journal. A few, like Latrobe, did die; some, like Buttrick, almost perished; and others, like Flint, quit the Valley until health was restored. Most of those who recovered wrote with postconvalescent reverence about their sicknesses. Mrs. Trollope, who "fell low before the monster that is forever strolling through that land of lakes

[26] Thomas, "Travels Through the Western Country," *Indiana Travelers,* 95, 119; Adlard Welby, *A Visit to North America and the English Settlements in Illinois,* in Thwaites' *Early Western Travels,* XII, 258; Henry R. Schoolcraft, *Personal Memoirs of a Residence of Thirty Years with the Indian Tribes,* 183; Wyeth, *Oregon, Early Western Travels,* XXI, 105.

[27] Quoted in Dorothy Anne Dondore, *The Prairie and the Making of Middle America,* 243–44.

and rivers, breathing fever and death," was typical of those who were relieved and grateful to have escaped almost certain death.[28]

Interestingly enough, travelers found few settlers willing to admit the unhealthy nature of their localities and issued warnings to their readers to be cautious of local testimonials. James Flint could not recall "having more than two persons acknowledge that they lived in an unhealthy situation." At Pittsburgh he was told that Marietta and Steubenville were sickly; at those places the people indicted Chillicothe. At Chillicothe the climate of Cincinnati was deprecated, and at Cincinnati many of the people were willing to transfer the greater menace to the falls of the Ohio River. Finally, at the falls, the truth was partially admitted, but it was affirmed that the Illinois country was even less healthy. Amos Andrew Parker had similar experiences at Detroit, Monroe, and Chicago. The same illusion (if not deceit) carried even into smaller areas. William Oliver, stopping along a small Illinois river, asked a resident if his settlement was healthy. Upon being assured that it was, he inquired about health on the opposite bank. "Well," his informer drawled, "guess it's full of ague . . . 'taint fit for nothing but a bull frog or a half-breed Frenchman." On the opposite shore he heard similar testimony, with the indictment reversed.[29]

Even in New Orleans there were those who felt that reports had been much exaggerated, that the city was far less unhealthy than was generally supposed. Harriet Martineau wrote of being handed a pamphlet, written by a physician, which denied "the

[28] John Bradbury, *Travels in the Interior of America*, 190; Schoolcraft, *Personal Memoirs*, 68–69; Benjamin Henry Boneval Latrobe, *Impressions Respecting New Orleans 1818–1820*, *xxiii*, 166n.; Tilly Buttrick, Jr., *Voyages, Travels and Discoveries*, in Thwaites' *Early Western Travels*, VIII, 54; John Ervin Kirkpatrick, *Timothy Flint: Pioneer, Missionary, Author, Editor*, 171; Frances Trollope, *Domestic Manners of the Americans*, I, 117.

[29] J. Flint, *Letters from America*, *Early Western Travels*, IX, 175; Parker, *Trip to the West*, 55; William Oliver, *Eight Months in Illinois*, 231–32.

unhealthiness of New Orleans as strenuously as some of its inhabitants deny its immorality." However, actions sometimes speak louder than words. For most of the inhabitants, the infectious summer seasons were periods to be feared and dreaded, and during those months an annual pilgrimage was made by those who could afford it to the highlands or to places of public resort. Latrobe noted that the principal merchants in New Orleans planned their business arrangements in order to be "at leisure about the commencement of July" so that they might flee the city, and he further noted that those who did so did not return "until the middle of October or the beginning of November." In 1832 alone, 15,000 of 50,000 residents fled the city to escape the double threat of cholera and yellow fever.[30]

Leaving an unhealthy location, temporarily or permanently, for a more wholesome one had been practiced rather extensively in Europe for several hundred years. The American residents along the Atlantic coast throughout the seventeenth and eighteenth centuries made frequent use of the technique as a means of escaping epidemic-ridden seaports.[31] And by 1820 it was firmly established in the minds of Valley residents that the only successful way to avoid or to cure diseases, medicine notwithstanding, was to seek a location or climate that was "above the fever line," sufficiently high to be free of the deadly effects of miasmata and fogs.

For temporary retreats, mineral springs, long the fashion in America and Europe, became popular throughout the Valley. Hardly an area was without one or more of these natural attrac-

[30] Harriet Martineau, *Retrospect of Western Travel,* I, 256–57; Edouard de Montule, *Travels in America 1816–17,* 96; Bullock, *A Sketch of a Journey Through the Western States, Early Western Travels,* XIX, 123; Duffy, *History of Medicine in Louisiana,* I, 140.

[31] Carl Bridenbaugh, "Baths and Watering Places of Colonial America," *The William and Mary Quarterly,* [3d series], Vol. III (April, 1946), 151–81; Fernand Engerand, "How Our Ancestors Spent Their Holidays," *Review of Reviews,* Vol. IX, (January, 1894), 85–86; Perrin du Lac, *Travel Through the Two Louisianas,* 7, 9.

tions, and as the demand for them rose many were commercially developed. Samuel Brown noted one in 1817 near Jeffersonville, Indiana, which had been "much frequented." Thomas Hulme, visiting Blue Licks (near present Paris), Kentucky, in 1818, described the mineral spring there as a "great resort in summer for the fashionable swallowers of mineral waters, the three or four taverns at this time completely crowded." The Yellow Springs near Dayton were described in 1832 by Timothy Flint as "the most accustomed watering-place" in Ohio, but he suggested that their "elevated position, the grand and romantic scenery, and the cool and salubrious air" probably contributed as much to the restoration of invalids as did the waters.[32]

Elevation and mineral or hot springs were the important elements in establishing the reputation of two of middle America's most celebrated health resorts, both of which rose to prominence during the first half of the nineteenth century. White Sulphur Springs, located high in the mountains of West Virginia, became a resort as early as 1788, and by 1833 was rated second only to the great Saratoga Springs in New York among American spas. Harriet Martineau, herself a bather, in 1837 noted that the springs were a resort for hundreds of patients who came with a variety of diseases "from a distance of 1,000 miles in every direction."[33]

Hot Springs, located high in the mountains of Arkansas, was another prominent resort. According to legend, the curative properties of these springs were known to Indians long before the first Europeans explored them. Just when they were first used by Americans has not been determined, but the springs were already in moderate use when Hunter and Dunbar visited them in 1804.[34]

[32] Samuel R. Brown, "The Western Gazetteer; or Emigrant's Directory," in Lindley's *Indiana Travelers,* 157; Thomas Hulme, *A Journal Made During a Tour in the Western Countries of America,* in Thwaites' *Early Western Travelers,* X, 68; T. Flint, *History . . . of the Mississippi Valley,* I, 403.

[33] Hoffman, *A Winter in the West,* II, 292; Martineau, *Society in America,* 184.

[34] An extract from William Dunbar's journal read: "At the hot springs they

Dr. Edwin James recorded in 1820 that there were in proximity to the springs some "twenty or thirty huts" which were used "at some seasons of the year by persons who resort hither for the benefit of the waters." Timothy Flint declared in 1832 that the springs were "a great and increasing resort for invalids from the lower country," and in the same year Congress, inspired by the increasing popularity and the undoubted (but at the time inexplicable) alleviating powers of the hot springs, set aside the lands embracing the numerous warm and mineral springs as a federal reserve. Hot Springs eventually became the oldest of the United States national parks.[35]

Some settlers, unable to afford prolonged periods of nonproductivity, made permanent adjustments by retracing their steps into the older settled areas. Thomas Nuttall met several persons in 1818 near Georgetown, Pennsylvania, returning from the western country "in search of a situation which might afford them health." William Faux near the Ohio River in 1819 passed five or six huge wagons laden with goods and families, "attended by horsemen, cattle, and footmen, and many negroes, all returning from the Missouri territory to . . . Kentucky . . . being scared out of Missouri by sickness." And William Forster, traveling near Vincennes, Indiana, in 1821 noted that there was considerable traffic on the roads, "some going out to Illinois and Missouri and nearly as many returning to their former residences, discouraged by sickness . . . ."[36]

---

found an open log cabin, and a few huts of split boards, all calculated for summer encampment, and which had been erected by persons resorting to the springs for the recovery of their health." [Thomas Jefferson], *Message from the President of the United States Communicating Discoveries Made . . . by Captains Lewis and Clark, Doctor Sibley, and Mr. Dunbar,* 105.

[35] E. James, *Account of an Expedition, Early Western Travels,* XVIII, 48; T. Flint, *History . . . of the Mississippi Valley,* I, 283; William Edward Fitch, *Mineral Waters of the United States and American Spas,* 219.

[36] Thomas Nuttall, *A Journal of Travels into the Arkansas Territory,* in Thwaites' *Early Western Travels,* XIII, 49; William Faux, "Memorable Days in

Still other pioneers, unwilling to give up their search for an Elysium, manifested a sincere interest in Texas following its opening to Anglo settlement in 1821. The Stephen F. Austin Papers are full of letters from residents in all parts of the Mississippi Valley, and conspicuous by association in their inquiries are questions relating to quality of the land and conditions of health. From Ohio came a letter stating, "The enquiries of my friends are directed principally to price and quality of land . . . and *the climate with regard to health*"; from Kentucky, "Is it a Rich and Healthy Country possesed of the advantages of Navigation"; from Tennessee, "I fear that I shall not have good health in this Country, and have but little doubt that in a part judiciously chosen in the Brassos that I should be healthy"; from Missouri, "I would Remark if the Country proves Healthy, I am destined for that section next fall"; from Arkansas, "The people of this country have been somewhat sickly. . . . Many will remove to Texas if they are not descouraged by some thing unseen"; and from Mississippi. "If accounts [of Texas] are flattering there will be considerable moving on as it is thought to be a healthy Climate and good soil for Cultivation."[37]

Thus by 1820 a trend in the continuing waves of western emigration was well established. The attractiveness of the "Promised Land" beyond the Mississippi Valley was determined not only by fresh soils but by their freedom from the fevers of the Valley as well; the quest for healthy locations and for health itself became important factors in determining population movements. Indeed, the prospects of finding a disease-free environment among western lands became the ultimate hope of a large reservoir of health-seekers whose constitutions were shattered by residence in the Valley of tombs.

America," in Lindley's *Indiana Travels,* 295; William Forster, "Memoirs of William Forster," *ibid.,* 257.

[37] Eugene C. Barker (ed.), *The Austin Papers,* I, 459, 522, 1489, 461, 689, 889 (citations are in order of reference above).

Moving westward after 1825 was not particularly easy; the official United States policy of concentrating civilized Indian tribes along and beyond the 95th meridian made expansion not only difficult but in many cases unlawful, and the myth of the Great American Desert left much of the plains region unattractive and unwanted. Nor was western migration for a majority of Valley residents especially desirable. Considerations of economic necessity forced many to risk exposure to the less desirable attending conditions, and a typical American characteristic, compulsive naïveté, gave many a pioneering soul a feeling of indestructibility, a special feeling of personal immunity from the endemic and epidemic diseases of the Valley. Thus, despite its extreme insalubrity, the Mississippi Basin filled rapidly with hopeful settlers.

There was, for instance, the hope that improvements incident to the advancement of civilization—land clearance, swamp drainage, and pest control—would bring relief to the Valley dwellers as it had to coastal residents in an earlier period; and there was always the hope that some new development would come in the treatment and cure of the prevalent diseases. In the latter aspiration, Americans everywhere were to be sorely disappointed; regrettably, scientific advancement throughout the century brought few improvements in medical practice, and Valley residents were forced to fight against their inanimate foes without much relief.

II. *The Dilemma of Nineteenth-Century Medicine*

MEDICAL SCIENCE during the century of westward expansion was an inevitable and tragic failure, inevitable because it was based on an erroneous philosophy, tragic because it offered but few dependable protections or reliefs from myriad terrifying diseases. Dependence upon false premises left physicians with an imperfect understanding of causal factors and relegated these men to a pragmatic and often desperate search for remedies.[1] Ineffective treatments robbed them of respect and prestige and invited an assorted collection of medical impostors into the profession. By mid-century the truth of the failure of formal medicine was admitted, and increasingly, doctors as well as pioneers placed a greater reliance upon change of residence and travel as a means of relieving illness or of escaping an infested location.

Medical science in the eighteenth and nineteenth centuries was a stepchild of the Enlightenment. The same rational idealism which insisted upon balanced equations, an ordered universe, and inalienable rights sent clinicians off on an unfruitful search for the causes of diseases in imbalanced natural forces. As such, medical theories became overwhelmingly oriented toward the dangers of "the epidemic constitution of the atmosphere," a mias-

[1] Oliver Wendell Holmes, *Medical Essays 1842–1882*, 195.

matic concept of contagion so confusing that medical progress was retarded for two centuries.[2]

The damaging obsession with miasmata was not an inexorable consequence of the new age of science; indeed by 1700 the rational groundwork had been laid for a sound theory of germ contagion, a theory developed in the sixteenth century by the Veronese physician Hieronymus Fracastorius and one only slightly at variance with modern concepts. No outstanding clinician emerged, however, to carry on his excellent beginning, and scientific discoveries during the period that followed had little effect upon the practice of medicine. Most of the nineteenth century physicians knew of dependable medication for but two of the many prevailing diseases—quinine for malaria and Jenner's vaccination for smallpox.[3] It was not until the growth of bacteriological science in the late nineteenth and early twentieth century that medicine was pried loose from its paralyzing theory of miasmatic contagion.

That outstanding members of the American medical faculty were gripped by the miasmatic theory is evidenced only too graphically in their writings. Dr. Benjamin Rush, most prominent of early American physicians, wrote in 1799 that "disease is the offspring of putrid vegetable and animal exhalation, . . . [and] filth acted upon by a hot sun in a *moist* state." He later classified the sources of dangerous miasmata as those arising from twenty-seven vegetable and eight animal-matter exhalations, some of which are as amusing as they are tragic. Among those vegetable in origin he listed putrid vapors arising from marshes, spoiled vegetables (especially cabbage, potatoes, pepper, Indian meal, and onions), the canvas of an old tent, old books and paper money that "had been wetted and confined in close rooms," and weeds which had been cut down and exposed to heat and mois-

[2] Charles-Edward Amory Winslow, *The Conquest of Epidemic Disease*, 161.
[3] Richard Harrison Shryock, *Medicine and Society in America 1660–1860*, 161.

ture near a house. Among those animal in nature he listed effluvia arising from human bodies left unburied, whales thrown upon the seashore, rawhides confined in stores, fish entrails, and privy wastes. Dr. Jabez Heustis, surgeon general of the United States Army in 1817, also believed "it a fact confirmed" that diseases were occasioned, among other things, by bad air and miasmatic exhalations arising from swampy situations. Still a half-century later, Dr. Austin Flint, author of a widely consulted textbook on the practice of medicine, acknowledged the putrid-vapor thesis. He wrote that endemics (diseases known to prevail within circumscribed territorial limits) "must be caused by poisonous miasmas [which] emanate from the soil," and that epidemics (diseases rapidly spreading or widely prevalent) were a product of the same miasmata which "must be diffused through the atmosphere." Even as late as 1888, Dr. W. C. Van Bibber noted that "the greatest number, as well as the most serious diseases, produced by the quality of the air alone, are found to originate in the lower strata of the air—that is, at an elevation but little above the level of the sea."[4] Thus, by a persistent compounding of an erroneous theory of contagion, the causes of disease remained unsolved mysteries for most of the nineteenth century.

Because existing knowledge of external causation (etiology) was imperfect, other vital areas of medical technique were seriously affected. Without an effective etiology, it was impossible to develop a permanent classification (nosology) of diseases, and without a reliable nosology, it was impossible to understand or diagnose even the elementary forms of sicknesses. Fevers, for

[4] Benjamin Rush, M.D., *Observations Upon the Origin of the Malignant Bilious, or Yellow Fever,* 4; Rush, *An Inquiry into the Various Sources . . . of Summer and Autumnal Disease in the United States,* 5–11; Heustis, *Physical Observations . . . of Louisiana,* 50, 57; Austin Flint, M.D., *A Treatise on the Principles and Practice of Medicine,* 106; W. C. Van Bibber, M.D., "The Therapeutic Value of Some of the Mineral Waters of the United States," *Transactions of the American Climatological Association,* Vol. V, (1888), 237.

example, frequently were regarded and treated as primary diseases themselves, not as symptoms of deeper distresses. Indeed, Daniel Drake, a leading Valley physician in the mid-nineteenth century, classified them under "Febrile Diseases: autumnal, bilious, intermittent, remittent, congestive, miasmatic, malarial, marsh, malignant, chill-fever, ague, fever and ague, dumb ague, and lastly *the* fever."[5] It is evident from Drake's list that to cure a fever was to relieve but a part of a patient's illness. Such inconclusiveness was generally characteristic of early medical practices.

Medical practice in the early nineteenth century was almost unbelievably primitive and ineffective. Illness too often resulted in death, or even more often in some permanent disability or disfigurement, despite the persistent efforts of dedicated medical men. Treatment of patients was based for the most part on the humoral doctrine, one that regarded internal causation or bodily susceptibility as arising from an imbalance of body humors such as blood, bile, lymph, and other body liquids. To make matters even worse, there was a sharp disagreement among trained physicians over the proper interpretation of the humoral doctrine. A more numerous "heroic" or orthodox fraternity of allopaths felt that the proper way to restore health to a patient was "to let blood out of him." Violent diseases, they believed, could be expelled only by violent practices or by medicines which produced actions in the body opposite to those accompanying the disease. Dysenteric patients, for example, were fed repeated doses of an emetic to induce vomiting. A smaller but highly vocal group of mild or botanic homeopaths advocated the use of herb teas, vegetable preparations, or steam-induced sweatings as a means of stimulating the natural restorative functions of a temporarily imbalanced system.[6]

[5] A. Flint, *A Treatise . . . of Medicine,* 127, 133; Shryock, *Medicine . . . in America 1660–1860,* 50; Drake, *A Systematic Treatise,* 703.

[6] Shryock, *Medicine . . . in America 1660–1860,* 51; Thomas Low Nichols,

Although there was persistent opposition to such harsh or heroic treatments, a majority of doctors bled their patients copiously (for almost every known disease) and prescribed powerful drugs in an effort to purge bodies of unwanted humors. Bloodletting was a terrifying experience for the patient; it was accomplished by severing a blood vessel with a lancet, by drawing blood through small perforations in the skin with crude suction cups, or by applying leeches directly to the patient's body. Purging was accomplished either by giving such drugs as calomel, castor oil, and mercury to induce purgation, or by administering emetic preparations such as tartar, ipecac, or opium to induce vomiting and sweating. "Bleed and purge" treatments actually killed many patients who could not stand the shock or the violent convulsions which accompanied them; still other patients were left too weak to ward off more serious infections.[7]

The distrust and fear which heroic practices aroused in the minds of the public cost the orthodox medical profession valuable prestige and many clients. Heroic medicine was, in a word, untrustworthy, and its inadequacies occasioned the rise of even greater chaos. Less courageous and disillusioned patients turned in increasing numbers to untrained quacks whose medicines and practices were at least more encouraging if not more efficacious.

It was difficult even for writers of that day to distinguish between regular and irregular practitioners. A diploma was easily obtained, and often none was needed. There were virtually no effective governmental regulations and there was a significant shortage of standardizing medical boards and certifying agencies. All practitioners, trained or untrained, were called "doctor." Thus attempts at classification were vague and meaningless except to those who defended one system over another. A partial list of

M.D., *Forty Years of American Life 1821–1861*, 226; Eugene H. Rosenboom and Francis P. Weisenburger, *A History of Ohio*, 127.

[7] William Ransom Hogan, *The Texas Republic: A Social and Economic History*, 232.

classifications left by a contemporary physician included allopaths, homeopaths, hydropaths, chrono-thermalists, Thompsonians, Mesmerists, herbalists, Indian doctors, clairvoyants, and spiritualists—each representing a distinct system of practice.

The conflict between many systems resulted in virtually no system at all; there was no clearly defined standard, no real science of medicine, no absolute or acknowledged authority. "One can scarcely conceive," a physician wrote in 1864, "of an honourable profession reduced to a lower ebb than that of medicine in the United States."[8]

The Mississippi Valley, more than any other section of America, tended to magnify the worst features of nineteenth-century medicine. Disease was so prevalent and the demand for doctors of any kind so great that almost anyone was allowed to practice. Thus the problem of frontier medicine was not one of quantity but of quality of practitioners, there being "many desperate and unprincipled quacks" for every trained physician.[9]

The skilled practitioner was truly a rarity along the frontier, not so much because competent physicians feared that they might be overworked or unappreciated as because they had the understandable desire to be paid for their services. Since there was seldom enough money for necessities and practically none for medical assistance, frontier doctors generally were homespun, self-taught products of the areas in which they resided.[10] Their formal training consisted of nothing more than reading a manual on practical medicine, and usually the pertinent section of the manual only at the precise moment it was needed to treat a patient. When book remedies failed, as they often did, the less responsible practitioner resorted to treatments of his own impro-

[8] T. L. Nichols, *Forty Years of American Life,* 225, 227.

[9] Edgar W. Martin, *The Standard of Living in 1860,* 227; Oliver, *Eight Months in Illinois,* 130.

[10] William Bollaert, *William Bollaert's Texas,* 300–301; Martin, *The Standard of Living in 1860,* 229; Hogan, *The Texas Republic,* 238.

vising. One traveler who fell victim to yellow fever in New Orleans in 1832 submitted himself to an untrained Frenchman who prescribed repeated doses of castor oil over a period of several days. In a single day, the traveler consumed four wine glasses of the highly purgative liquid. The operation of the medicine was "not one way, but every way," and he imagined that he "would have no insides left to go home with." Remarkably enough, he survived both the treatment and the fever, and he rather good naturedly, but somewhat unconvincingly, recommended the castor oil treatment to others with similar ailments.[11]

Men of every conceivable persuasion and calling were attracted to the healing arts, and settlers in western communities often suffered as much from the "contradictory systems of the swarm of medical men" as they did from "the pestilential exhalations of the surrounding marshes."[12] These irregular doctors, who depicted heroic practitioners as butchers who went about armed with lancets, denounced all orthodox methods, yet borrowed liberally from them whenever it became expedient. For this reason no reliable classification of quacks has been devised. Perhaps the one left by Dr. Willis King in 1891 is as useful as any: grouping them into four categories, he listed gentlemanly quacks, smart pretenders, professional buzzards, and advertising quacks. The gentlemanly quack was capable but willfully ignorant of *materia medica*; the pretender was a loudmouthed know-it-all whose failures frequently compelled him to abandon a community in order to escape the wrath of duped patients; the buzzard was a "dismal old fraud" who dispensed time-honored but harmless herb teas and vegetable preparations; and the advertising quack, guarantor of elaborate and expensive wonder cures for the worst kinds of diseases, was a "cunning, cruel . . . thief, a cowardly robber and a merciless pirate, a murderer and a vil-

[11] Wyeth, *Oregon, Early Western Travels,* XXI, 95.
[12] Giacomo Constantino Beltrami, *A Pilgrimage in Europe and America,* 79.

lain so black and damnable" that the English language "fails to furnish words with which to paint him."[13]

To this list should be added a group of supernaturalists—spiritualists, clairvoyants, phrenologists, and the like, whose special forte was cancer and other incurable diseases. Reputed to possess unusual healing powers, these men placed less stress upon medicines and more on miracles and superstitions. Although they employed many strange and mysterious techniques, they often did nothing more than look a patient over somberly, lay a hand on him, and read a favorite verse from the Scriptures. Few of the incurably ill ever recovered, but if one in a thousand of those who visited a "faith healer" did so, it was enough to establish the reputation of the "doctor" forever. Many zealous and disease-ridden Christians found it extremely difficult to resist the wiles of smooth-talking, Bible-quoting frontier parsons who also dabbled in the art of healing.

If a disrespect for orthodox doctors occasioned the growth of unorthodox practitioners, a distrust of heroic, "puke and purge" medicines promoted a susceptibility for packaged nostrums or patented medicines, the demand for which became almost a national mania. Quack medicines, for the most part, were not medicines at all but were cleverly disguised, well-advertised elements of a nefarious business enterprise. Unscrupulous nostrum manufacturers fought like vultures over a steadily increasing market for their fraudulent panaceas, and fortunes were made from the manufacture and sale of "sarsaparilla, pills, bitters, cough elixers, cures for consumption, etc." A box of pills which cost a penny to make sold for a quarter; one costing a quarter sold for a dollar. Quinine, the best of the available fever fighters, sold anywhere from six to thirty dollars an ounce. And whenever a nostrum acquired a reputation for itself, hosts of imitations were

[13] Willis P. King, M.D., *Stories of a Country Doctor*, 122, 381–85; see also an interesting editorial: "Quack Medicine Advertisements," *The Medical and Surgical Reporter*, Vol. LI (November 29, 1884), 627–28.

produced by rival companies in an effort to capitalize upon its popularity, resulting in a constantly overcrowded market.[14]

Quack doctors and apothecaries dispensed scores of preparations without much discretion, and credulous and ignorant people swallowed them voluminously at the first recognizable sign of sickness. Opium preparations, frequently prescribed in small amounts as pain killers by orthodox physicians, were sold so indiscriminately in western towns that at least one entire community became addicted to the drug. The same was true of bitters (medicinal liquors), which were intended only to soothe internal irritations but provided instead an easy avenue to alcoholism for many who used them to excess.[15]

No discussion of patent medicines would be complete without reference to the elaborate claims made by their manufacturers. Perhaps one example will serve the purpose of a hundred: Doctor Hoofland's *Celebrated German Bitters*, for instance, were advertised as an effective cure for

> liver complaint, dyspepsia, jaundice, chronic or nervous debility, diseases of the kidneys, and all diseases arising from a disordered liver or stomach, such as constipation, inward piles, fullness of blood to the head, acidity of the stomach, nausea, heartburn, disgust for food, fullness or weight in the stomach, sour eructations, sinking or fluttering at the pit of the stomach, swimming of the head, hurried and difficult breathing, fluttering at the heart, choking or suffocating sensations when in a lying posture, dimness of vision, dots or webs before the sight, fever and dull pain in the

14 Milo Milton Quaife (ed.), *Pictures of Gold Rush California*, 63; Gustav Dresel, *Gustav Dresel's Houston Journal: Adventures in North America and Texas, 1837–1841*, 105; see also Stewart H. Holbrook, *The Golden Age of Quackery;* Nichols, *Forty Years of American Life*, 227; Pickard and Buley, *The Midwest Pioneer*, 108. The practice of trademark copying led inevitably to court action; at least one case ultimately reached the United States Supreme Court. See: *Manhattan Medicine Company* v. *Woods and Another*, 108 U.S. 218 (1882). For a reaction by the medical profession to this case see "Patent Medicine Suits," *The Medical and Surgical Reporter*, Vol. LI (July 26, 1884), 101–102.

15 Holmes unfortunately failed to identify the town. Holmes, *Medical Essays*, 200; Nichols, *Forty Years of American Life*, 227.

> head, deficiency of perspiration, yellowness of the skin and eyes, pain in the side, back, chest, limbs, etc., sudden flushes of heat, burning in the flesh, constant imaginings of evil, and greai depression of spirit.[16]

Interestingly enough, quackery was defended, even promoted, by the very people it victimized. Many ordinary men felt that the "plain man of common sense [was] superior to the trained expert" and persistently resisted all efforts to curb the practices of quacks or to restrict the sale of nostrums, the consensus being that such limitations did violence to the spirit of equalitarianism and freedom so characteristic of the "age of the common man." "Thus," a prominent medical historian has summarized, "did Jacksonian Democrats proclaim their inalienable rights to life, liberty, and quackery."[17]

Quackery also was bitterly attacked, although such protests fell on unresponsive ears for a time. Professional men were "hard on quacks, and rightly so," for what they regarded as a wanton disregard for ethics and standards, but their efforts were rendered impotent largely because of the limited effectiveness of their own practices. Similarly their attacks on quack medicines, the *materia medica* "which consists of sugar of milk and a nomenclature," were useless because pillmakers had "a constituency of millions"—the public "which insists on being poisoned."[18] And all too frequently it was the irregular, not the regular, doctor who emerged from the controversy with the better reputation despite

16 Advertisement in the *Texas Almanac for 1857*.

17 Shryock, *Medicine . . . in America 1660–1860*, 149. For an excellent study on this subject see James Harvey Young, "American Medical Quackery in the Age of the Common Man," *Mississippi Valley Historical Review*, Vol. XLVII (March, 1961), 579–93.

18 "Professional Quacks," *The Medical and Surgical Reporter* Vol. LI (November 29, 1884), 697; Shryock, *Medicine . . . in America 1660–1860*, 148; Holmes, *Medical Essays*, 186. Apparently, quackery continues to be a menace to American society; see especially: American Medical Association, *National Congress on Medical Quackery, October 6–7, 1961*.

the support given to trained physicians by powerful organs of public opinion.

Newspapers consistently made a whipping post of unorthodox practitioners in an attempt to expose the baseness of their practices. Typical of the editorials which dealt with this subject are these:

> Texas is about as full of quacks as McKinney's Bayou is of ducks. As we have no time to go shooting the latter, we have a half notion to amuse ourselves by exposing the disreputable practices of the former. There is many a doctor in Texas who has no other sheepskin than his own good-for-nothing hide.

And:

> The medical profession will never regain the position it once held in the public estimation, and to which it is entitled, until the colleges cease to throw out upon the world such numbers of "half baked saw-bones." When the possession of a diploma shall become evidence that the holder is an educated gentleman, then will the doctors be honored as they ought to be. But when, as at present two out of every five in the profession are neither doctors nor gentlemen, the profession, as a body, cannot claim that which otherwise belongs to it. A whole bale of sheepskins cannot transform a quack into a physician.[19]

Medical impostors also were made the brunt of many lighthearted but meaningful satires. *Harper's Weekly* in a regular column called "Things Wise and Otherwise" rarely omitted a sarcastic stab at quackery, such as these barbs:

> "Doctor Kalorum, do you think my darter will get well?"
>
> "Well, if she don't get no wuss, and does get some better, she may probably get over it. That is my opinion, madam, and I think I ort to know."

And:

> "I suppose," said a quack, while feeling the pulse of a patient, "that you think me a humbug."

[19] Galveston *News*, January 17, 1871; August 21, 1872.

"Sir," replied the sick man, "I perceive you can discover a man's thoughts by his pulse."[20]

No part of this verbal war obscured for very long the knowledge that formal medicine was a colossal failure. Proof that western homesteaders recognized this fact rests in the great reliance which was placed upon folk cures and home remedies. Most adults were well acquainted with the symptoms of the more common diseases and had some homespun method of treating each of them.[21] Many families refused to call in a doctor until all household remedies had been applied without effect or unless there was an emergency.

Domestic medicine to a great extent was "a combination of homemade science, empiricism, and superstition."[22] As much faith was placed in domestic preparations made from natural ingredients such as barks, roots, catnip, slippery elm, saffron, and various noxious vegetables and weeds, as in marketed products such as quinine, calomel, spirits of niter, castor oil, paregoric, laudanum, alum, and liniments. Few families, however, were without both types of medicine, and some member of the family, often the woman of the house, was responsible for keeping a ready supply on hand and was assigned the task, usually by default, of dosing afflicted members of the family.

Another essential aid for household treatment was a handbook of medical recipes and practices which was consulted as often for the relief of the body as the Scriptures were for the soul. Handbooks prepared and sold by doctors invariably reflected the particular bias of their authors, but in the absence of a more reliable authority, the suggested treatments were merely added to favored home remedies and were then religiously applied. "My

20 "Things Wise and Otherwise," *Harper's Weekly Magazine,* January 3, 1857, p. 14; May 2, 1857, p. 286.

21 E. James, *Account of an Expedition, Early Western Travels,* XVII, 84; Martin, *Standard of Living in 1860,* 232.

22 Pickard and Buley, *The Midwest Pioneer,* 35.

folks," one writer asserted, "had one of Dr. Gunn's family doctor books, and it recommended gun powder (black powder, of course) and sweet milk for snake bite. That was all they gave me, and [then] put a 'stingy green' tobacco poultice on my foot." Typical of the books prepared by the laity was Mary S. Bosley's *Hand-book on Useful Knowledge, Comprising a Valuable Selection of Recipes in Medicine, Choice Things in Cookery, New Ideas in Gardening, etc., etc.*[23] In an amusing way, those who purchased a standard medical text instead of Mrs. Bosley's *Hand-book* appear to have been cheated somewhat by comparison.

Prepared drugs were usually administered in their purchased form, although at times so injudiciously as to occasion much grief; natural ingredients were compounded into a variety of teas, elixirs, poultices, pills, and powders. Alcohol, when available, was a favorite mixing additive for orally consumed medicines, but spring, well, and river water was also used. Mineral water, as previously noted, was always highly prized and was sometimes taken in lieu of domestic medicines. Some pioneers believed devoutly in the efficacy of the murky waters of the Mississippi and Missouri rivers. Henry Schoolcraft, suffering from a severe liver ailment, traveled several miles to drink the "turbid, but healthy waters" of the Mississippi, and returned to his station "in completely restored health." And many Missourians believed firmly in the healthful properties of their "Big Muddy," a river described as "a little too thick to swim in and not quite thick enough to walk on," and they considered pure water from Rocky Mountain streams downright unhealthy because of its clearness.[24]

[23] Solomon Alexander Wright, *My Rambles as East Texas Cowboy, Hunter, Fisherman, Tie-Cutter*, 22. Dr. Gunn's *Domestic Medicine* also stated that "any man unless he was a fool or an idiot, could amputate an arm or leg, provided he had a half a dozen men to hold the victim down." Quoted in Duffy, *History of Medicine in Louisiana*, II, 57; Mary S. Bosley (ed.), *Hand-Book of Useful Knowledge*, 3ff.

[24] Schoolcraft, *Personal Memoirs*, 12; Grantley F. Berkeley, *The English Sportsman in the Western Prairies*, 141; Richardson, *Beyond the Mississippi*, 19.

Faith in muddy water undoubtedly stemmed from the folk superstitions which played such a vital role in western medicine. These superstitions were expressed in a number of ways. There was a widespread belief that anything nauseous and noxious was good for the sick, and domestic medicines were esteemed in proportion to their bitterness and potency. To cite specific illnesses, a sore throat might be cured by tying around the neck at bedtime a stocking which had been worn during the day, rheumatism by wearing a rattlesnake skin around the waist, and ague by wearing pulverized rock salt in stockings. Additionally, the virtues attributed to teas prepared from certain barks were determined by the manner in which the bark was stripped from trees; if the bark was peeled upward, the tea acted as an emetic, and if peeled downward, it induced purgation.[25] Finally this humorous bit of superstition needs little clarification:

> The women even blamed certain makes of wagons for carrying certain diseases. One mother said, "My Georgie Anne is much healthier than Ollie. You know, Mrs. Allison, my Georgie Anne was born in a *Shuttler*. My Zeke traded it for a *Studebaker* to Ike Johnson, and that wagon is sure great for every epidemic or itch, or measles that comes along. Then Zeke traded the *Studebaker* for a *Bain*, and my kids got the mumps in that wagon. Give me a *Shuttler* any day for healthy kids, Arabella."[26]

The varieties of folk cures for any particular illness stagger the imagination. For example the ague, "like hard work a concomitant of the frontier," was treated with such things as strong teas made from barks and combined with "large draughts of whiskey"; elixirs made from boiled sassafras roots; pills made from quinine, calomel, steel dust, cobwebs, and black pepper;

[25] Holmes, *Medical Essays*, 187–88; King, *Stories of a Country Doctor*, 126, 129; Bosley, *Hand-Book of Useful Knowledge*, 37. Robert Fowler, an early fur trapper, cured a sore throat by applying "a sock [filled] with ashes" around his neck. *The Journal of Jacob Fowler*, 127; Pickard and Buley, *The Midwest Pioneer*, 40 n., 42, 129.

[26] James A. McKenna, *Black Range Tales*, 161.

and blister plasters made of mustard or Spanish fly. Even sagebrush, the only vegetation on the arid plains, was regarded as useless except that "when used as a medicine, it [was] a specific for ague." There were treatments even more novel. John Gladwyn Jebb, a western traveler humbled by ague, disdained "taking quinine by the pailful," stripped off his clothing, and chased away his fever by sitting neck deep in the cool water of a stream. And W. H. Ryus effected an "ague-cure" by removing his clothes, burying all but his head in a shallow ditch, and sleeping "all night in the Mother Earth." A partially relieved Ryus completed his cure with a three-month tour of the prairies during which he gained forty pounds and "never had another chill."[27]

If as a general rule there was but casual agreement among the precursors of orthodox, quack, and domestic medicines on the treatment of diseases, there was one ague-cure among those listed above on which there was almost universal accord—Ryus' extended tour of the western plains. His journey, though not precedent-making itself, was a prototype of a widely used method of treating many kinds of afflictions. Traveling for health was not new to mid-nineteenth-century Americans; physicians in both Europe and America had for a long time been aware of the beneficial effects of prolonged journeys or changes of residence even for diseases considered incurable. Such treatments, however, were expensive and inconvenient and were prescribed in most cases for the more affluent or as a last resort for the incurably ill.[28]

[27] E. James, *Account of an Expedition, Early Western Travels*, XVII, 84; Buley, *The Old Northwest*, I, 246; Pickard and Buley, *The Midwest Pioneer*, 111; W. F. Rae, *Westward by Rail: The New Route to the East*, 91; Mrs. John G. Jebb, *A Strange Career: Life and Adventures of John Gladwyn Jebb*, 111–12; W. H. Ryus, *The Second William Penn: A True Account of Incidents that Happened Along the Old Santa Fe Trail in the Sixties*, 12.

[28] For a detailed description of favored European tours for health written by the Physician Extraordinary to the King of England, see James Johnson, M.D., *Change of Air, or the Pursuit of Health; an Autumnal Excursion through France, Switzerland, and Italy, in the Year 1829*.

If men of medicine displayed some reluctance in utilizing the travel-cure technique, it is understandable; each person dispatched on a sea or land voyage represented another admission of the failure of medical knowledge. Yet conscientious physicians were not prone to delude themselves by meaningless rhetoric; they were only too aware of their own personal failings and those of formal medicine. "Every practical physician," wrote Daniel Drake at mid-century, "is aware of the frequent failure of all kinds of medication . . . and of the great value of cool and fresh air . . . united with active exercise, simple diet, new scenery, and the disuse of all medicine." Austin Flint stated that if other measures failed to relieve a patient, "nothing is to be depended on but a change of residence." And William Gerhard added that for lingering illnesses and especially consumption, "nothing is so efficacious as a journey, with its necessary consequences, a change of air."[29] Thus nineteenth-century medicine bowed once more at the feet of Nature, the god of the Enlightenment, but in so doing it discovered a shrine around which physicians everywhere could unite. Travel for health became the panacea which early medicine could not supply, and with increasing gusto the medical fraternity endorsed the practice and accepted Nature as a full partner in the art of healing.

Two types of therapeutic travel generally were prescribed. For patients needing absolute rest, sea voyages during favorable seasons of the year were highly recommended. Invigorating sea air, simple ship's diet, and restricted deck life often worked wonders on debilitated constitutions—provided voyages were long enough to permit gradual convalescence. "A short voyage is of little comparative benefit," Dr. Gerhard conjectured; "hence, one to the East Indies, or to the Mediterranean, or to South America answers best."[30] There was a major drawback, however, to this type

[29] Drake, *A Systematic Treatise,* 397; A. Flint, *A Treatise . . . of Medicine,* 231; William Wood Gerhard, M.D., *Lectures on the . . . Diseases of the Chest,* 52.
[30] *Ibid.,* 112

of treatment; water travel was quite expensive and was "totally beyond the reach" of many patients. As a result the greater number were obliged to resort to prolonged land journeys.

Overland travel, especially for residents of the Mississippi Valley, generally was the surest means of dissipating an incipient illness and of insuring restoration to complete health. It was also the chief hope of those who sought to escape the source areas of endemic diseases during the sickly summer months. Land trips were necessarily attended with greater inconveniences, but the invalid traveler could expect the same refreshing change of air and plain chuck-wagon fare. Greater physical exertions were inevitable, but to many doctors increased activity as a therapeutic agent was as highly regarded as a purer atmosphere. "Driving, riding, walking, gunning, fishing, boating, bathing, yachting, or botanizing . . . if used wisely and in moderation," Dr. Bushrod James wrote, "will stimulate the functions of the respiratory and digestive organs and skin, and prove generally beneficial in effect." Dr. Gerhard advised similarly: "If the strength of the patient is good, the journey should be made on horseback, or in an open carriage, and be pursued as long as the strength of the patient continues to improve."[31]

Of all the land routes available to those seeking a temporary or permanent change of residence, the ones which gained the widest reputation in the nineteenth century were those which extended across the western prairies and plains. The disease-free and health-restoring environment of the "Great American Desert," discovered by early pioneers long before the medical profession recognized it as such, had become quite celebrated by the late 1830's among patients and doctors for its sanative effects.[32]

By 1850 even "the most important medical figure of his age in America" subscribed wholeheartedly to what he termed "Jour-

[31] Bushrod W. James, M.D., *American Resorts: with Notes Upon Their Climate,* 155–56; Gerhard, *Lectures on the . . . Diseases of the Chest,* 112.

[32] Josiah Gregg, *Commerce of the Prairies* (ed. by Max L. Moorhead), 23.

neys of Health on the Great Plains." Daniel Drake, most picturesque of the pioneer physicians in the Mississippi Valley, grew up in Kentucky, studied and taught in Ohio medical schools, and practiced his profession in many parts of the Valley. As an orthodox physician by training and conviction, he embraced both the miasmatic and heroic philosophies of medical practice, but as a humanitarian, he had a sympathetic interest in his patients which kept him alert to fresh ideas and promising innovations. He also was a gifted writer with a style suggestive of Mark Twain, and he entertained and educated Valley residents over a period of several years.[33]

Easily the most valuable and influential of Drake's literary output was the magnificent *Diseases of the Interior Valley of North America*, a forty-year record and synthesis of early American medicine which he published in 1850. Throughout its several hundred pages, the book reveals repeatedly how great a disciple of fresh air and therapeutic travel he had become in the declining years of his practice. Like so many of his contemporaries, Dr. Drake had great concern for the large number of Valley residents who were incapable of becoming acclimated to their surroundings, those who showed an excessive susceptibility to recurrent attacks of autumnal diseases. His frank appraisal was that "as long as they continue in an infested locality, the [fevers] will set all the efforts of [medicine] at defiance. Change of place must, then, be submitted to, or the constitution will be ruined." Special attention, he felt, should be given to finding a location where fevers were not endemic, an end which could be accomplished among other ways by "wandering in the desert west of the Mississippi."

[33] Donald T. Atkinson, *Magic, Myth and Medicine,* 232; Drake, *A Systematic Treatise,* 174; Drake, *Discourse on the History, Character and Prospects of the West,* unnumbered introductory pages. For Drake's most humorous work see his posthumously published, *Pioneer Life in Kentucky: A Series of Reminiscential Letters.*

He listed three "recognized routes" by which invalids might traverse the arid plains, a voyage up the middle Missouri River, a tramp along the overland route to Oregon, or a journey down the trails to Santa Fe.[34] Of the three, a trip up the Missouri was the least regarded because "the opportunity for making a distant voyage on this river [did] not often occur." Changes of latitude and elevation, however, and the novelty and wildness of the scenery made such a summer voyage pleasant and invigorating, but Drake advised that "it should not be preferred to the others, by any who have health and strength to travel by land." A trip to Oregon was much more advantageous. Although the journey was long and the terrain varied, beyond the 100th meridian fevers were seldom to be met with and dews were so inconsiderable "that but little inconvenience is felt from lodging on the grass, even without a tent." Invalids, he felt certain, would find such journeys to be of "radically curative and reinvigorating influence."

Drake reserved his highest praise for the most southerly route, the trail to Santa Fe. Only one disadvantage—a much warmer climate—detracted from the many advantages which this route held over the others. The surface traveled across did not generate autumnal fevers, the road was open for a longer period each year, and the distance, though definitely of sufficient length, was not so great as that to Oregon or northern California. In addition, an invalid, if he desired, had the prerogative of extending his journey by "descending the valley of the Rio del Norte to the luscious vineyards of the El Paso, or [ascending] to the rich and beautiful valley of Taos and thence [scaling] the surrounding outliers of the Rocky Mountains."

The doctor concluded his discussion of these routes with an estimate of their therapeutic values. He recognized that each abounded in exposures, fatigues, and privations but held the view that such inconveniences were precisely what made the trips

[34] Drake, *A Systematic Treatise;* the summary may be found on pp. 174–75.

beneficial. "Take them away," he wrote, "and a journey over the desert to the Rocky Mountains would be scarcely more efficacious than the fashionable voyage to Europe."

For what types of diseases were the plains routes recommended? "Every enlightened physician will answer," he retorted, for all forms of dyspepsia, even that depending on chronic gastritis; chronic disorders of the liver, spleen, and bowels; morbid sensibility and morbid imagination, including every shade of hysteria and hypochondriasis; apoplexy in its incipient stage, and lingering and partial palsies; haemoptysis (spitting and coughing of blood usually resulting from hemorrhages in the lungs) and tubercular consumption in every stage.

Thus it seems clear that the medical fraternity had reached a degree of frustration somewhat analogous to that which haunted the midwestern pioneer; if the pioneer could not find health in the Valley, his doctors could not guarantee him relief if he remained there. Invalided settlers had no alternative except to travel, doctors none other than to encourage them to do so at the earliest opportunity.

III. *Paths of Hope to a Frontier of "Perfect" Health, 1820-40*

UNTIL 1820, few obstacles other than fevers and Indians slowed the pace of the persistent western emigrant who surged into and out of the various frontier towns, exuding confidence and enthusiasm for whatever lay over the next horizon. Then, almost as if the frontier had moved too rapidly, the West was beyond Independence, Missouri. There, for the first time, the line of settlement which had moved so rapidly from Pittsburgh to Chillicothe, Cincinnati, Louisville, and St. Louis came to an abrupt halt.

Independence, from its founding in 1827 until the Civil War, was the gateway to a new experience in western penetration. Nothing in the previous pattern of settlement had prepared pioneers for the treeless, arid plains which stretched before them, nor had they encountered the Indians so concentrated or hostile. Accordingly, unobstructed settlement of western lands virtually was suspended for three or four decades, and the Plains and Rockies frontier became one for individuals not the masses, for adventure not homesteading, and for quick exploitation not patient development. This was a blow not only to agriculturalists but also to those who desperately needed to leave the Valley for reasons of health. Thus the health-seeker and the healthful western climate came together only under the most difficult of circumstances.

Unconscious greatness and unparalleled ignominy awaited the plains and mountain pioneer. Brave men struck out into the uncertain wilds of remote western regions and became legendary heroes while performing the simplest of tasks for the basest of motives; but as if guided by some great equalizing force, intrepid trappers built up—then exhausted—a lucrative trade in furs; enterprising entrepreneurs reached—then deluged—Santa Fe with profitable trade goods; and adventurous Argonauts discovered —then squandered—fortunes in mineral wealth. By mid-century only the miner found a persistent attraction at a time when the exploits of the other groups were fast becoming the deeds of yesterday.

The legends which surround these early adventurers have been so romanticized that it is customary to study the New West in the light of their interests and achievements; the discerning student feels almost obligated to retrace each trail step by step, to recount the furs pelt by pelt, or to reweigh the gold ounce by ounce. These were, admittedly, the West's lowest common denominators, but the West was more than roads, beavers, and bonanzas.

Submerged beneath the glamorous exploits of trappers, traders, and Argonauts is a fully documented, but until recently ignored, group who were as adventurous as and perhaps even more courageous than the other groups mentioned.[1] The men in this group were known by various names in the literature of the West, but they were most frequently identified as "health-seekers." Referred to rather inconsistently as lungers, consumptives, phthisics, coughers, hackers, invalids, valetudinarians, sanitarians, asthmatics, rheumatics, white plaguers, pukers, and walking death, many of them were the silent but ever present partners of

[1] John E. Baur, "The Health Seeker in the Westward Movement, 1830–1900," *Mississippi Valley Historical Review*, Vol. XLVI (June, 1959) 91–110; see also his *The Health Seekers of Southern California, 1870–1900.*

the better-known trail blazers. They were, for the most part, frustrated Valley residents, driven to travel either in a desperate attempt to cure a diseased body or as a means of escaping contamination.

Perhaps the consignment of the health-seeker to relative obscurity is justifiable, perhaps not. Certainly it is not true that his contributions were less spectacular or less fundamental to the development of the West than those of his more publicized contemporary; indeed, invalids were present at least in supporting roles at every stage of frontier development. Even more important, many of the more famous personalities were health-seekers before they became frontier heroes. And ironically, it was the invalid's frontier that remained as a prominent western attraction long after all other frontiers had lost their appeal.

The health frontier did not develop suddenly; it arose gradually from the accumulated experiences and reports of western travelers and did not achieve definite dimensions for more than half a century. Some part of the health legend which surrounded it dates to the earliest days of Spanish occupation; one account in 1773, for instance, indicates that "no diseases have appeared since the settlement of the province [New Mexico] by the Spaniards, which can be said to be peculiar to the climate and country. The seasoning or bilious fever is only known in the country south of the 30th degree of latitude."[2] However, most of the reliable information (printed or circulated in English) on the healthfulness of western regions was obtained after the official explorations of the Louisiana Territory began.

If the collection of meaningful data began with the Lewis and Clark Expedition in 1804, much of the material relating to health in their journals is rather ephemeral. Their journey was not attended with a freedom from infections; a Sergeant Charles Floyd

[2] Frederick Webb Hodge (ed.), "A Virginian in New Mexico in 1773–74," *New Mexico Historical Review*, Vol. IV (July, 1929), 249.

died of "bilious cholic," and the entire company was sometimes "troubled with mild dysentery." On the whole, however, the general health of the party was "quite good, if not better than that of the same number of men in any other situation" despite the absence of many conveniences and the exposure to extremes in weather.[3]

Potentially the most influential feature of this expedition is found not in the official journals but in the personal experiences of Meriwether Lewis. Captain Lewis had from childhood been subject to "hypochondriac affections . . . a constitutional disposition in all the nearer branches of the family." His condition had on occasion caused his family considerable alarm, but Lewis managed to control the disorder most of the time. During his western expedition, the constant exertions of body and mind "suspended these distressing affections," and he enjoyed a brief period of grateful relief.[4] His respite was temporary, however, for upon his return to sedentary life in St. Louis, the old symptoms "returned with double vigour," and he grew steadily worse until he met a strange death (probably suicide) a few years later in a small Tennessee town. Captain Lewis unknowingly became the first American health-seeker to tour the trans-Mississippi West, but it is improbable that his brief recovery in the plains and mountains had a substantial effect upon the budding health legend.

Zebulon Pike's reflections on health factors along the prairies and mountains in 1806 were equally laconic, though he also mentioned infrequent attacks of fever, rheumatism, and frostbite among his men. His chief contributions to health statistics arise from a generous estimate of the air and climate of New Mexico

[3] Paul Allen (ed.), *History of the Expedition under the Command of Captains Lewis and Clark,* 30, 48.

[4] Thomas Jefferson, "Life of Captain Lewis," biographical introduction to Paul Allen (ed.), *History of the Expedition . . . of Captains Lewis and Clark, xxi–xxii.*

and Texas and from an occasional reference to a medicinal or warm spring along his route.[5]

The early journalists must be excused for their failure to elaborate on most subjects, for boldness, brevity, and a hasty departure were characteristic of all things military in the age of exploration. Some of the later army accounts are somewhat more informative, but after 1820, it should be recalled, the deplorable conditions of the Mississippi Valley were so well known that even military men were noticing the great contrast in health between Valley and Plains residents. The journals detailing Stephen Long's 1819–20 expedition, for example, are of some value in this regard:

> [The Indian's] catalogue of diseases, and morbid affections, is infinitely less extensive than that of civilized men. Rheumatism is rare, and gout appears to be unknown. No case of phthisis or jaundice fell under our observation. . . . They are rarely afflicted with dysentery . . . [and] are never known to be subject to [sunstroke], although they travel for days and even weeks over the unsheltered prairies. . . . Fevers, and fevers and ague, are exceedingly rare.[6]

Long's expedition was the last of its type for over twenty years, and by 1840 many of the health attractions of the trans-Mississippi West had become well known. It is not surprising, therefore, to find John C. Frémont reporting in 1842 that "the climate [on the plains] has been found very favorable to the restoration of health, particularly in cases of consumption."[7] Nevertheless,

[5] Zebulon Montgomery Pike, *The Expeditions of Zebulon Montgomery Pike,* II, 362, 424, 597–600, 728, 779.

[6] E. James, *Account of an Expedition, Early Western Travels,* XV, 43–44. The Indian suffered more from the white man's diseases than from those native to his habitat, but this fact appears not to have caused too great a conscience stricture among desperate and unprincipled emigrants. George Catlin, for example, wrote in 1841 that six million Indians had fallen victim to smallpox. *Letters and Notes of the Manners, Customs, and Conditions of the North American Indians,* I, 6.

[7] John C. Frémont, *Report of the Exploring Expedition to the Rocky Mountains in the Year 1842, and to Oregon and North California in the Years 1843–44,* 49. For evidence of the influence of this report on the public, see Eliza Greatorex, *Summer Etchings in Colorado,* 6–9.

the reports of these earlier military explorers played a substantial role in establishing or confirming the West's reputation for healthfulness; perhaps no greater evidence of this fact can be offered than the following statement written by Daniel Drake in 1850:

> From what can be collected out of the travels and expeditions of Lewis and Clark, Pike, Long, Catlin, Fremont, and Gregg, not less than from fur traders and Santa Fe Merchants, [autumnal fever] is almost unknown at the distance of three hundred miles from the western boundary of the states of Missouri and Iowa.[8]

Thus, most of the work of forging a health legend was accomplished between 1820 and 1840. From Drake's testimonial it is possible to identify many of the people who contributed to its building, and certainly the fur trappers and Santa Fe merchants are the two groups most responsible. One other source bears mentioning, however, one with which Drake undoubtedly was familiar and one which was quite influential in the southern regions of the Mississippi Valley.

If Drake read thoroughly his home-town Cincinnati *Literary Gazette* on June 12, 1824, he could not have missed this letter describing the Comanche Indians in Texas:

> Providence seems to have provided them with some natural indemnities against the physical evils. . . . incidental to their irregular and versatile manner of life. . . . They are subject to few diseases, and exhibit many instances of remarkable longevity. . . . The almost unqualified salubrity of the climate they occupy, certainly has a large share in this unusual prolongation of life and activity.[9]

The letter was the last in a series of four written for the *Gazette*

[8] Drake, *A Systematic Treatise*, 704.

[9] "David G. Burnet's Letters Describing the Comanche Indians," with an Introduction by Ernest Wallace, West Texas Historical Association *Year Book*, Vol. XXX, (October, 1954), 138–39.

by David G. Burnet, onetime Cincinnati resident turned Natchitoches merchant.

Burnet's story is one of surprising successes. Afflicted with what apparently was a terminal case of pulmonary consumption, he abandoned his mercantile operations in Louisiana in 1817 on the advice of his physician and crossed into Texas, which at the time was largely uninhabited and under alien control. He sought out the Comanches near the headwaters of the Colorado and lived with them according to their customs for more than a year. "The food, exercise, and climate of the . . . region repaired the wastes of disease, renewed his physical energies, and restored him to vigorous health."[10]

A restored Burnet established permanent residence in Texas in 1826, served with distinction throughout the early Texas rebellion, and became ad interim president of the republic in 1836. Because his destiny was so intimately blended with that of Texas, the story of his recovery grew more important as he became more prominent. Burnet's search for health among the Plains Indians must rank among the very earliest of its type, and many people presently followed in his footsteps.[11]

Important though Burnet's experiences were to Texas immigration, they were soon overshadowed by a large volume of reports from fur trappers and Santa Fe merchants attesting to the restorative qualities of the upper Plains and Rockies region. Each of these groups rose to prominence after 1820, and each made an extremely valuable contribution to the western health legend.

After the turn of the nineteenth century, almost a generation

[10] Jacob De Cordova, *Texas: Her Resources and Her Public Men,* 158; A. M. Hobby, "Life of David G. Burnet," *Texas Almanac for 1873,* 159.

[11] Burnet's search for health was well known among early Texans. Austin, in recommending him to his Mexican superiors in 1826, described Burnet as one to whom *"el clima frio de Ohio no era favorable a su salud."* Eugene C. Barker (ed.), *The Austin Papers,* II, 1349; A. B. Lawrence, *Texas in 1840: Emigrant's Guide to the New Republic,* 103.

passed before the American fur trade grew out of its trial and error stage. Only a few hardy adventurers during that time taunted their British-Canadian rivals and probed into the secrets of Rocky Mountain regions, and although Washington Irving records that the overland Astorians returned to St. Louis in 1813 "in perfect health and fine spirits," most of the early reports are spotty and inconclusive on the subject of health.[12]

It was not until the year 1820, about the time of Long's expedition, that trapping and trading became a permanent and important factor in developing the western country. Hundreds of men thereafter left Missouri towns annually in the service of newly formed fur companies and returned after each season to squander a year's booty and to spread their illustrious tales. Among stories, both printed and verbal, of extreme privation, intense loneliness, and extended danger, were mingled accounts of the proverbial salubrity of the remote West. In time, these simple testimonials were compounded into a full-blown health legend.

Mountain men were amazed but happy to find the western country so healthful. William H. Ashley, co-founder of the Rocky Mountain Fur Company, recorded in 1825:

> I have not known at any time a single instance of bilious fever among them [trappers] or any other disease prevalent in the settled parts of our country, except a few instances (and but very few) of slight fevers produced by colds or rheumatic affections . . . . Nor have we in the whole four years lost a single man by death except those who came to their end prematurely by being either shot or drowned.[13]

Similarly, a statement attributed to the firm of Smith, Jackson and Sublette around 1830 noted that "among our partisans in the

[12] Washington Irving, *Astoria; or Anecdotes of an Enterprise Beyond the Rocky Mountains,* I, 249.

[13] Harrison Clifford Dale (ed.), *The Ashley-Smith Explorations,* 135.

mountains, sickness and natural deaths are almost unknown."[14] Kit Carson, "a symbol of the best and bravest of the far western frontiersmen," asserted that the happiest days of his life were spent among the trappers in the wonderfully healthy air of the mountains:

> Notwithstanding . . . hardships and irregular habits, sickness was absolutely unknown among us. I lived ten years in the mountains, with from one to three hundred trappers, and I can not remember that, during the whole period, a single one of them ever died from disease.[15]

And George Catlin, celebrated artist and author who traveled extensively throughout the 1830's among the American Indians, frequently met and traveled with "hundreds of mountain men who . . . lived exactly upon the Indians' system, continually exposed to the open air . . . and, to all the disappointments and privations peculiar to that mode of life." He concluded that he "never saw a more hardy and healthy race of men in [his] life whilst they remain in the country."[16]

To these declarations can be added the weight of the personal experiences of trappers who themselves benefited from the sanative qualities of chilled mountain atmosphere. All of the Sublette brothers, especially William and Andrew, had the "taint of consumption in their blood," and were driven to mountain life partially as a means of combating the disease.[17] Robert Campbell, a clerk after 1832 for Ashley and William Sublette, made several trips into the mountains "mostly on account of his health." W. T. Hamilton, whose constitution had been undermined by chills and

[14] Hiram Martin Chittenden, *The American Fur Trade of the Far West,* I, 66n.

[15] Richardson, *Our New States and Territories,* 10.

[16] Catlin, *Letters and Notes,* II, 228.

[17] Frank Triplett, *Conquering the Wilderness,* 496; LeRoy R. Hafen, "Mountain Men—Andrew W. Sublette," *The Colorado Magazine,* Vol. X, (September, 1933), 180. William Sublette almost perished from tuberculosis in 1834 while traveling in the Rockies and did die of the disease in 1845 at Pittsburgh, "far from his beloved mountains." John E. Sunder, *Bill Sublette, Mountain Man,* 128–29, 230.

fevers, entered into partnership with Bill Williams in 1842 and became a mountain trader in an effort to rid himself of a lingering cough. And there is some evidence that Charles Larpenteur, from whose pen came "the most valuable contemporary document extant" on the fur trade, also suffered from ill health. Finally, Antoine Robidoux, who like most Missourians knew firsthand of the ravages of fevers and ague, left the Valley in 1824 and became a prominent trapper in the Colorado (western) River area in the twenty years that followed.[18]

Although many details of his active life are missing, Robidoux nonetheless offers the best example of how, by word of mouth, the health legend was disseminated among frontier folk. His travels took him to many parts of the Far West, but of all places visited he reserved his keenest appreciation for California, the "perfect paradise." His glowing discussion of that place before an assemblage in Missouri in 1840 greatly influenced the organization of the first overland party to California. According to John Bidwell's account of the meeting, Robidoux answered "every conceivable question" put to him. "Generally," Bidwell remarked, "the first question a Missourian asked about a country was whether there was any fever and ague." He continued:

> I remember his answer distinctly. He said there was but one man in California that had ever had a chill there, and it was a matter of so much wonderment to the people of Monterey that they went eighteen miles into the country to see him shake.[19]

For a land which Robidoux had already described as "one of perennial spring and boundless fertility," nothing could have

[18] Charles Larpenteur, *Forty Years a Fur Trader on the Upper Missouri,* I, 8, *xxii*; William T. Hamilton, *My Sixty Years on the Plains,* 18; Dr. Benjamin Harrison, son of President William Henry Harrison, joined Larpenteur in his 1833 trip to the Rockies in an effort to break himself of a habitual thirst for whisky. Joseph J. Hill, "Antoine Robidoux, Kingpin in the Colorado River Fur Trade, 1824–1844," *The Colorado Magazine,* Vol. VII (July, 1930), 125.

[19] Joseph Williams, *The Joseph Williams Tour,* as reprinted in LeRoy R. and Ann W. Hafen (eds.), *The Far West and Rockies Historical Series, 1820–1875,* III, 200; John Bidwell, *Echoes of the Past about California,* 14.

excited his audience more than his pleasing remarks on its healthfulness.

When fur trappers were not persuading men to travel into the salubrious Rockies on their own, some were guiding parties of health-seekers there themselves. Andrew Sublette enjoys the distinction of having led the first of such parties into the mountains. His own health in 1844 had grown suddenly worse; he had "a persistent cough and wanted to return to the mountains for his health."[20] Almost providentially the opportunity came in the spring of that year when a group of twenty men, eleven of whom were traveling for their health, persuaded him to act as guide for the westbound party. He led them to the northwestern part of Colorado, to Brown's Hole on the Green River, where some of the invalids improved rapidly. Sublette himself enjoyed a return to such good health that he did not want to leave the country; nevertheless, by October, 1845, Sublette, much improved in health, was back in Missouri with fifteen of his party.

Thus, the western country came to be known for its remarkable climate, and as Hiram Chittenden has concluded, mountain men "loved it for its healthfulness."[21] Enforced abstinence "kept the body well and the mind clear. If starvation often stared the hunter in the face, the disorders of an over-fed stomach never disturbed his slumbers nor sapped his constitution with disease." The hunter found nature in perfect equilibrium, perhaps not so much for the hopeful homesteader as for the adventurous trapper and the desperately ill.

Of equal importance in the development of the West's reputation for health were traders of a different sort; Santa Fe merchants, for the most part, traveled in covered wagons and not on pack mules, crossed arid prairie lands instead of chilled mountain ranges, and sought Mexican specie rather than beaver skins.

20 LeRoy R. Hafen, "Colorado Mountain Men," *The Colorado Magazine*, Vol. XXX (January, 1953), 20; Sunder, *Bill Sublette*, 225.

21 Chittenden, *The American Fur Trade*, I, 660.

The New Mexican trade began with sporadic and perilous contacts during the last few decades of Spanish rule, but long years of restraint on such trade ended with the successful Mexican revolution in 1821. The flow of American-made goods thereafter became as welcome to New Mexican residents as it was lucrative for Missouri merchants.

With the official opening of Mexican-American relations, Missouri, entrepôt for both the fur and Santa Fe trade, became a center of business activity and attracted scores of enterprising merchants and adventurous muleteers. A line of towns directly along the Missouri River developed swiftly; older settlements such as St. Louis and Franklin received a fresh stimulus, and newer towns such as Independence and Westport sprang into existence near the western boundary of the state. And in 1825 the powerful Senator Thomas H. Benton persuaded Congress to mark off and to provide a military escort for an official road which linked Missouri and New Mexico trading centers.

Unhappily for the growth of this trade, the lands in Missouri, very much a part of the Mississippi Valley, proved to be extremely unhealthy; fevers and ague were so prevalent that Missourians were nicknamed the "Pukes" by the same pioneers who dubbed Ohioans "Buckeyes," Indianans "Hoosiers," Michiganders "Wolverines," and Illinoisians "Suckers."[22] Many people died annually from autumnal disorders; still others "vomited forth" from the state in search of a more salubrious area. By the 1830's each western terminus became a collecting point for invalids whose hearts were set upon exacting not material but physical rewards from a trip across the plains and prairies.[23]

Upon cursory examination, the Santa Fe Trail hardly seems an appropriate route for invalids to take. From Independence and Council Grove to the Cimarron Crossing (near the 100th

[22] A. Parker, *Trip to the West and Texas,* 86–87; Richardson, *Beyond the Mississippi,* 132.

[23] Gregg, *Commerce of the Prairies* (ed. by Moorhead), 23.

meridian) on the Arkansas River, travelers were still below the fever line and were therefore subject to endemic infections. Accounts are legion of those who suffered severely from these disorders during the first two hundred miles of their journeys; even William Becknell, to whom the credit is given for opening the Santa Fe trade, reported after crossing the Osage River in Kansas that nearly all of his men were sick "and much discouraged."[24] At the Cimarron Crossing, where the road forked, the threat of fever diminished, but dangers of a different sort awaited the traveler. Along the southern route (Cimarron Desert cutoff) water was sometimes so scarce that it was necessary to cut open the stomachs of buffalo in order to obtain that life-sustaining liquid, and along the more extended western route (Turquoise or Raton Pass cutoff) lack of water was no threat to survival, but fierce Plains Indians were—just as they were in any part of the plains region.

A closer examination, however, indicates that a number of advantages accrued to the health-seeker who took either of these routes to Santa Fe. Military organization of each wagon train reduced the danger of Indian raids considerably; the warm (often hot) plains sun baked health and strength into debilitated bodies; and the pure, invigorating prairie air soothed and restored diseased lungs. More important, invalids who might resort to a southwestern jaunt were not limited to those who had sufficient strength to walk or ride horseback; indeed, a considerable number who were totally incapacitated began their journeys bedfast in one of the many wagons in each caravan or in a specially equipped carriage. The slow, easy pace of a three months' trip to Santa Fe permitted the valetudinarian to convalesce at his own pace.

The greatest reward actually came at trail's end; all who reached New Mexico were in agreement that such towns as Santa

[24] Archer Butler Hulbert (ed.), *Southwest on the Turquoise Trail,* 57.

Fe and Taos possessed "very agreeable climates." While on an unauthorized trading venture, a desperately ill Virginian was brought to Santa Fe after his capture by Spanish officials. The climate of the city "greatly aided in [his] recovery—the air . . . being dry, pure and bracing." And he added:

> I feel from my experience at Santa Fe, that the chances of life are considerably more in our favour there than in the most healthy parts of the continent east of the Rocky Mountains. Colds . . . never prove fatal without the greatest neglect. The seasons are mild and agreeable, the atmosphere constantly pure and elastic; and the sky clear, unclouded and brilliant.[25]

This report, if reputable, represents the experiences of the first Anglo-American known to have recovered from ill health in that region of the West; he did not, however, reach Santa Fe via the overland trails but by the Río Grande. Exactly when the Santa Fe road was first used by a health-seeker is not known since none of the earlier journals of New Mexican traders are very helpful in this regard. The first record of this route is that of General George C. Sibley, one of three commissioners authorized by Congress in 1825 to survey an official trade route to Santa Fe.

A descendant of an old and distinguished New England family, Sibley entered government service in 1805 at the newly established Indian trading post of Fort Bellefontaine near St. Louis. He was reassigned in 1808 to Fort Osage on the Missouri River, and from this post he was commissioned to assist in surveying the road to Santa Fe.

General Sibley accepted the proposed assignment with some reluctance. Writing to another of the commissioners, Benjamin H. Reeves, in 1825, Sibley remarked:

> For my own part I feel most sensibly that I have embarked in a service that will be found extremely arduous & in many particu-

[25] F. W. Hodge (ed.), "A Virginian in New Mexico in 1773–74," *New Mexico Historical Review,* Vol. IV (July, 1929), 249.

> lars extremely unpleasant; that I shall necessarily make sacrifices of time, interest, comfort, & perhaps health . . . not to be compensated by the pay allowed me. I will go on however without looking back; and if God gives me health and power, I will . . . do all in my power to make it useful to the country & honorable to those concerned in it.[26]

The concern he displayed for his health played a significant role in his decision to join the expedition. On May 1, 1825, he wrote to Owen Simpson in St. Louis: "A principal reason for my entering upon this duty is the hope and belief that it may be beneficial to my health, which tho' not exactly *bad* at this time, is [and] has been for 3 or 4 years indifferent." Sibley apparently suffered from recurring attacks of bilious fever which, in the course of time, had weakened him considerably, and although he was hopeful that western climates would strengthen his body, he actually was not sure that he would return from the perilous adventure.[27]

He began the journey on June 27, 1825, "quite unwell, with strong bilious symptoms" and frequently alluded to his ill health thereafter until September 22, when he recorded that all in the party were "in good health and fine spirits." At Santa Fe, he was again indisposed because of fatigue and severe headaches, but at Taos on March 26, 1826, he recorded in his diary: "Since my return from S[an]ta Fee, I have got entirely well again, and am now in as good health as I ever was."[28]

Sibley, upon his return to Missouri, lived a long and active life, reaching the age of eighty. Although it is doubtful that more than a handful of people knew of his quest for health on the prairies, his experiences inadvertently influenced the life of perhaps the most renowned invalid associated with the early health frontier—Josiah Gregg, pale-faced merchant of the Santa Fe trade and man of many talents.

26 *The Road to Santa Fe: The Journal and Diaries of George Champlin Sibley*, 222.

27 *Ibid.*, 31, 216.

28 *Ibid.*, 50 ff., 84, 141, 158.

Few men earned a greater reputation than Gregg in the development of the early West. His biography reads like a great adventure novel, and it is difficult to believe that so many activities were the experiences of a single individual.[29] Gregg was, in chronological order, a surveyor, teacher, lawyer, Santa Fe merchant, trail blazer, mule trader, author, soldier, physician, scientist, gold-seeker, and explorer. The list might even have been longer had not complications resulting from a riding accident terminated his life on February 25, 1850, at the age of forty-four. Yet, Gregg embarked on his multifarious career in a most humble way as a hopeless invalid, apparently destined for a consumptive's early grave but grimly determined to exhaust every possibility which offered some hope of restoring his rapidly declining health.

No stranger to frontier life, he was born in Tennessee in 1806, and moved with his parents, Harmon and Suzannah Gregg, first to Illinois and then to Missouri, a pattern of movement often duplicated by those caught up in the early westward surge. Though he inherited his parents' spirit of adventure, Josiah was obliged to follow a more sedentary existence, for he was a delicate youth with definite symptoms of tuberculosis. His condition was further complicated in 1829 by attacks of chronic dyspepsia, and the serious illness he suffered during that year was but a prelude to even greater distresses; the following year his health failed completely, and he was confined to his chambers "for nearly a twelvemonth," his afflictions defying "every plan of treatment that the sagacity and science of [his] medical friends could devise."

So debilitated did his condition become that hope virtually was

[29] The biographical data which follow are drawn from two sources: Max L. Moorhead's "Introduction: the Author," in his edition of Gregg's *Commerce of the Prairies, xvii–xxix*; and Paul Horgan, "Josiah Gregg Himself," *Diary and Letters of Josiah Gregg*, I, 3–40; II, 3–30.

abandoned for his recovery. Although he had the best of available medical attention, his doctors in a final gesture admitted their failures and advised him as a last resort to join a Santa Fe–bound wagon train for a trip across the prairies. Such advice might have seemed incongruous to almost anyone but Gregg; most men in his hopeless condition would have preferred the few conveniences available in frontier settlements to the life of a prairie tramp.

Gregg, nevertheless, made preparations to join Jesse Sutton's trading caravan scheduled to depart from Independence for Santa Fe in May, 1831. The decision to do so was prompted in part by the numerous stories of miraculous prairie cures which circulated in every frontier community. Indeed, Gregg's knowledge of the health-restoring qualities of western climate was more than mere rumor; some members of his immediate family had firsthand experiences in crossing the arid plains. Milo Quaife suggests that Gregg's father may have been a participant in William Becknell's 1822 trading venture to Santa Fe.[30] Additionally, two of Josiah's brothers, Jacob and John, later made the overland trip to New Mexico at different times. Undoubtedly the most significant encouragement was that supplied by Jacob, who was a member of George Sibley's survey team in 1825 and who could attest to the improvement in the General's spirits and health during the expedition. Thus, fortified by both hearsay and fact, Josiah began his trip of desperation in an ambulance carriage especially equipped for his purposes.

The effect of prairie environment was phenomenal and his recovery rapid. Within a week he felt confident enough to ride horseback by day and to sleep in the open air by night; and a week later he was strong enough to hunt buffalo with the more robust of his companions. By the time he reached Santa Fe, he had traded his heart for his health; his handmaiden became the

[30] Gregg, *The Commerce of the Prairies* (ed. by Quaife), *xv*.

prairies, and he never again knew real happiness or felt quite well when absent from them. As he traveled back and forth on his eight trips across the prairies, Gregg became, along with the men who had preceded him, one of the living testimonials to the restorative qualities of plains and mountain environments. Because his experiences found their way into print, his influence greatly exceeded that of all the others combined.

His remarkable contribution to the development of a frontier for health in the West resulted from a penchant he had for keeping a statistical and descriptive record of his travels. Some of his experiences were published in the late 1830's in Arkansas and Texas newspapers, and in 1844 the full text of his notes became, with the aid of John Bigelow, the highly respected and widely circulated *Commerce of the Prairies.* Although it was intended primarily to narrate the experiences of Gregg's nine years as a merchant in the Santa Fe trade and as a resident of northern Mexico, the book became, in effect, the first major piece of promotional literature on the health attractions of the trans-Mississippi West to reach a nationwide audience.

For the medical profession, Gregg, himself a physician by 1846, became a recognized authority and his book a source of primary information. Dr. Daniel Drake was so impressed with the work that he quoted (in his *Diseases of the Interior Valley*) long passages from it in an effort to substantiate his own growing belief in the efficacy of the western climate.[31]

For the potential health-seeker, Gregg's book contained a wealth of encouraging testimony. At the outset he stated:

> For some months preceding the year 1831, my health had been declining under a complication of chronic diseases . . . my physicians advised me to take a trip across the Prairies, and in the change of air . . . to seek that health which their science had failed to bestow. I accepted their suggestion.[32]

31 Drake, *A Systematic Treatise,* 156.

32 Gregg, *Commerce of the Prairies,* (ed. by Moorhead), 3–4.

His readers thereafter were continually reminded that they were reading a remarkable success story, one that might be duplicated by any invalid with courage enough to follow in Gregg's footsteps. Moreover, Josiah's tantalizing descriptions of prairie environment must have made the urge to do so almost irrestible. "The *climate* of most parts of the Prairies," he wrote in one place, "is no doubt healthy in the extreme; for a purer atmosphere is hardly to be found." And in another:

> It is most usual to sleep out in the open air . . . for the serene sky of the Prairies affords the most agreeable and wholesome canopy. The deleterious attribute of night air and dews, so dangerous in other climates, is but little experienced upon the high plains; on the contrary, the serene evening air seems to affect the health rather favorably than otherwise. . . . During dry weather . . . even the invalid prefers the open air.[33]

For the desperate invalid encaged in the insalubrious Mississippi Basin, the greatest feeling of release was found in the contrasts he drew between the climates of New Mexico and the Valley:

> Salubrity of climate is decidely the most interesting feature in the character of New Mexico. Nowhere—not even under the much boasted Sicilian skies, can a purer or a more wholesome atmosphere be found. Bilious diseases—the great scourge of the valley of the Mississippi—are here almost unknown. . . . Persons withered almost to mummies, are to be encountered occasionally, whose extraordinary age is only to be inferred from their recollection of certain notable events which have taken place in times far remote.[34]

Such were the encouragements of Josiah Gregg, the most prominent of the early health-seekers.

The first few decades after 1840 were years of transition in the development of the West; wars and prospecting replaced

[33] *Ibid.*, 43, 363.
[34] *Ibid.*, 3–4.

trapping and trading as the chief stimuli in bringing men into the region. Yet, because of the groundwork laid by such men as the Sublettes, Robidoux, Sibley, and Gregg, no great distance or no amount of danger kept numerous invalids, perhaps broken in health but not in courage, from racing to each new bonanza or from accompanying any military campaign. Sick men climbed out of their valley of frustration and walked along paths of hope to the plains and mountains, and in so doing helped to establish with some degree of permanence the dimensions of the western health frontier.

IV. *Expanding the Nation and a Health Frontier, 1840-60*

THE TWO DECADES before the Civil War were dramatic, action-filled years in the development of the West. If brave men after 1820 pioneered the trails across plains and mountains, men of equal courage after 1840 embarked along the same paths to complete the course of empire and to exploit western mineral wealth.

Before 1846 the undisputed boundaries of the United States extended no farther west than the crest of the Rockies, but at the conclusion of the Treaty of Guadalupe Hidalgo in 1848, the American flag flew proudly over the Pacific Coast at all but the very apex of the nation's contiguous continental expansion. Acquisition in itself did not bring a rapid influx of settlers to these remote coastal regions, but Sierra Nevada gold did. The events which led up to the Mexican conflict and the subsequent discovery of precious metals in California were vital not only to the nation's expansion but to that of the health frontier as well. Some illumination of those events is therefore necessary in order to trace the growth of the western health legend.

As the attractiveness of some parts of the western country became more widely known after 1820, periodic ruptures occurred in the relatively static Michigan-Iowa-Missouri-Arkansas-Louisiana line of settlement. The first of these ruptures occurred in

1821 with Anglo migrations into Mexican-held Texas. Somewhat later, smaller groups worked their way overland to Oregon and California and established isolated communities of American settlers. In all of these settlements the search for health was a constant, if secondary, objective; in at least one of them—Texas—health-seekers played a prominent role in shaping the destiny not only of a local area but of the entire western country as well.

Among the concessions granted to American citizens, Mexican authorities regretted most their decision to permit Americans to settle in Texas, for this indomitable group proved to be the catalyst for the events of the fateful forties. The men who answered Stephen F. Austin's call to the Brazos bottoms did so for a variety of reasons, chief among which was cheap land, but all who came shared one thing in common—an Anglo heritage of unalienable individual rights and self-determined government. Significantly, this heritage was compatible with the Mexican constitution of 1824, a frame of government which had received the enthusiastic approval of all liberal and republican factions in the new Mexican Republic.

Fully satisfied with their status under this constitution, American settlers in general gave unrestrained loyalty to Mexico until Santa Anna and his turncoat Centralists abrogated the constitution and established a dictatorship. Thereafter, all of Mexico seethed with unrest, and several major rebellions (including the one in Texas) broke out, all of which were aimed at restoring the constitution of 1824. Texas, last of the areas of revolt to feel the wrath of an uncompromising Santa Anna, broke openly with the Centralist government and, in a surprising show of force and with an amazing amount of luck, defeated Santa Anna at San Jacinto in April, 1836.

Victory at San Jacinto brought only *de facto* independence and unending rumors of Mexican reprisals; Texans in an understandable search for security then sought speedy annexation by the United States, an aspiration vehemently opposed by a war-threatening Mexico. The possibility of annexation remained a constant irritant between Mexico and the United States until it became a fact; annexation then became the immediate cause of the Mexican War.

Standing prominently among the leaders of early Texas was a substantial number of former invalids. For them at least, the hope of renewed health was a primary consideration for removing to the state; once restored, they repaid their indebtedness to a salubrious Texas with valiant conduct during the revolution and faithful service to the republic and state. But because their heroic deeds were accomplished in a time of great tension, their earlier years as health-seekers have largely been forgotten.

It would not be too incorrect to assert that all, not just a prominent few, who came to Texas were health-seekers after a fashion, for it would have been the exception rather than the rule if any had escaped affliction by the prevailing Valley endemics. For this reason, there was a persistent interest in any description of the conditions of health and climate in Texas. Contemporary writers, casting a comparing eye toward fever-ridden neighboring localities, were almost singular in their praise of Texas' climate, although their frequent warnings against overexposure in particular locations or in the wrong season of the year injected a sufficient amount of reality and accuracy into their estimates.[1] Stephen Austin made this estimate:

> The climate of Texas I deem to be decidedly superior in point of health and salubrity to any portion of north America in the same parallel. The margins of our rivers in common with all rivers of the world are somewhat subject to fever and ague and other complaints incident to similar situations but I think that the practical experience of seven years justifies me in saying that the rivers of Texas are less liable to diseases than any river of the U. S. below

[1] Samuel Harman Lowrie, *Culture Conflict in Texas 1821–1835*, 26–27.

> latitude 36. Situations back from the rivers, or near the Coast, are remarkably healthy.[2]

Mary Austin Holley in 1836 added:

> While we claim nothing unreal, no poetic exaggeration, or fictitious excellence for this region, we could confidently assert that no state on the continent is more eminently favored by nature in fertility of soil and salubrity of climate than Texas or presents a like combination of natural advantages. . . . A strong point of difference between the climate of Texas to that of Louisiana . . . consists in the superior *dryness* of Texas.[3]

Summed up, the fairest description of all sections within Texas was written anonymously in 1837:

> Were I asked my opinion of the health of Texas, in a comparative point of view, I would say that the lower country, from the Trinity to the Colorado, is as sickly, to say the least of it, as the most unhealthy portions of Louisiana, that between the Trinity and Sabine, it is as salubrious as the healthiest parts of this state, and that west of the Colorado and from this river to the Rio de las Nueces, even down to the coast, no southern country is freer from disease. It might be added, . . . that the country becomes healthier at any point as you recede from gulf.[4]

These qualified affirmations, along with simple expediency, were the two factors most responsible for the migration to Texas of a steady stream of men who had grown despondent about their chances of survival in the disease-ridden Mississippi Basin. Among those who came for reasons of health before the revolution were such outstanding Texans as Benjamin R. Milam, Francis W. Johnson, Erastus (Deaf) Smith, Amasa Turner, Mirabeau B. Lamar, and Anson Jones, as well as ad interim President

[2] *The Austin Papers*, II, 166. For a similar description, see Stephen F. Austin, "Descriptions of Texas, 1828," *Southwestern Historical Quarterly*, Vol. XXVIII, 104.

[3] Mary Austin Holley, *Texas* [*1836*], 40–41.

[4] Andrew Forest Muir (ed.), *Texas in 1837: An Anonymous Contemporary Narrative*, 132.

David G. Burnet, who had found health on the Indian prairies some years earlier. In general, their recovery of health in the rejuvenating Texas climate prepared them for the heroic deeds from which they have derived well-deserved fame.

A companion of Burnet's during his Comanche sojourn was Benjamin R. Milam. A near-fatal siege of yellow fever drove Milam to Texas, but he was fully recovered and eager to fight when Texas joined the general rebellion against Santa Anna in October, 1835. Colonel Milam aided the liberal faction in Coahuila in an attempt to move the seat of government from Saltillo to San Antonio. The conspirators were caught by Centralist troops, but Milam escaped to Texas, where he joined the volunteer army. He was killed during the assault he led on the besieged city of San Antonio de Bexar in December, 1835.[5]

When Milam fell, another former invalid, Virginia-born and malaria-ridden Francis White Johnson, took command and led the Texans to victory and the capture of the Alamo.[6] Johnson, alleged to be Texas' earliest historian, lost much of the reputation he earned at Bexar following his involvement in the abortive Matamoros expedition later in December.

Also present at the siege of Bexar were Erastus "Deaf" Smith and Amasa Turner. Smith moved from Mississippi to Texas in 1821, recovered his health but not his hearing, and became the most trusted scout of the revolutionary forces. Turner emigrated from Alabama in 1833, quickly threw off an incipient disease, and participated with Robert M. Coleman's company in assaulting the Mission City.[7] Both thereafter endured patiently Houston's forced retreats throughout much of March and April, 1836, and both responded valiantly to the General's commands at San Jacinto on April 21. Smith, in a daring morning raid, destroyed

[5] Walter Prescott Webb (ed.), *The Handbook of Texas,* II, 191.

[6] *Ibid.,* I, 915.

[7] Andrew Jackson Sowell, *Heroes of Texas: Deaf Smith,* 1; W. P. Webb, *Handbook of Texas,* II, 622, 809.

Vince's bridge and sealed Santa Anna's fate. Turner, in the surprise afternoon assault, led a company of infantry which helped to rout and annihilate the enemy. Thus did health-seekers, perhaps with a cougher's handkerchief in one hand and a soldier's rifle in the other, crown themselves with glory during this most crucial battle.

As in battle during the revolution, so in service to the republic did former health-seekers respond to the challenge of leadership. Of the four men who served as presidents of the short-lived republic, three (David G. Burnet, Mirabeau B. Lamar, and Dr. Anson Jones) entered the state with diseased bodies, the lone exception being Houston, twice elected to the post, who arrived with a sickness of the soul rather than of the body.[8]

Lamar, second of the popularly elected presidents, came to Texas from Georgia in January, 1835, badly afflicted with tuberculosis, a disease which had claimed his wife a few years earlier.[9] He recovered rapidly and participated with distinction throughout the revolution, achieving the rank of colonel and the command of Houston's cavalry at San Jacinto. He served as vice-president during Houston's first administration and succeeded him as president in 1838.

Among the decisions Lamar made as president was one which led to the disastrous Texan–Santa Fe expedition in 1841. Believing the New Mexicans would welcome the opportunity to unite with the Lone Star Republic and desiring to divert some of the lucrative Santa Fe trade to Texas, President Lamar without the sanction of his congress encouraged an organized expedition

[8] Although Houston was not a health-seeker, some of his closest friends were, among them being Z. N. Morrell, an old Tennessee buddy and itinerant Baptist minister, and Hamilton Stuart, a staunch political defender and Galveston newspaper editor. Z. N. Morrell, *Flowers and Fruits in the Wilderness,* 21, 369; *The Writings of Sam Houston* (ed. by Amelia W. Williams and Eugene C. Barker), IV, 420–21.

[9] Asa Kyrus Christian, *Mirabeau Buonaparte Lamar,* 5.

to embark on what a critic called a "chase of silly hopes and fears, begun in folly, closed in tears."[10]

On a journey accompanied by many hazards, privations, and inconveniences, the presence of men with emaciated bodies may seem strange, but by 1841 men in poor health and with little hope of recovery were seizing any opportunity, no matter how bizarre the prospects, to travel across the vaunted prairies. Thus, word of Lamar's proposed New Mexican campaign spread quickly throughout Texas and Louisiana and attracted a large number of adventurers, merchants, Indian fighters, soldiers of fortune, and men seeking to cure an "inflamation of the lungs." Among those who sought a prairie cure were George Barnard, L. C. Blake, Franklin S. Coombs, George Wilkins Kendall, and G. H. Strain.[11]

Easily the most prominent of these men was Kendall, editor of the New Orleans *Picayune,* chronicler of the Santa Fe expedition, and famed war correspondent in the Mexican War. "In the early part of April, 1841," he wrote somewhat later, "I determined upon making a tour of some kind upon the great Western Prairies, induced by the hope of correcting a derangement of health." While weighing the attractions of the various routes, he met Major George T. Howard, "then in New Orleans purchasing goods for the Texas Santa Fe Expedition."[12]

With a newspaperman's love of a good story, he made his choice. But Kendall exercised poor judgment in electing to accompany the Texans, for he was taken into custody in New Mexico by Mexican officials along with his bedraggled, half-starved companions and forced to make the long, tortuous march through sand and dust to confinement in Mexico. That he survived the

[10] Quoted in George Wilkins Kendall, *Narrative of the Texan Santa Fe Expedition,* I, *xix.*

[11] Noel M. Loomis, *The Texan–Santa Fe Pioneers, xiv,* 204ff.

[12] Kendall, *Texan Santa Fe Expedition,* I, 3.

arduous trek was a remarkable feat for an invalid, but fortunately for the health legend, he not only survived but lived to write a history of the expedition, a record 40,000 copies of which sold in eight years, in which he added his own testimony to the efficacy of western climates.

A re-elected Houston replaced Lamar in 1841 on the heels of this tragic undertaking, and was himself succeeded in 1844 by Dr. Anson Jones, last president of the Texas Republic. During Jones's abbreviated tenure (he served but a little over one year of a three-year elective term), this famed regimental surgeon at the Battle of San Jacinto, who had entered Texas in 1834 badly debilitated by malaria, declared an end to the republic and witnessed its annexation to the United States in 1845.[13] Thus, a chapter in the history of Texas was closed, and most fittingly so, by the pale hands of a restored invalid.

News of the revolution in Texas, which bore some resemblance to the earlier American struggle with Great Britain, was read with avid interest throughout the United States. As a result Texas and Texans played their part in expanding the western health legend. Knowledge of the climatic advantages and of the experiences of restored coughers was easily noticeable within the texts of material describing the new nation. The Reverend Chester Newell, for example, told his readers that his *History of the Revolution* in Texas (1838) was written during a year's residence in Texas for his health.[14] And A. B. Lawrence's *Emigrant's Guide to the New Republic* (1840) included the following encouraging testimony:

> In the opinion of respectable physicians and others a residence in this country would be as likely to mitigate or relieve pulmonary and consumptive affections, as any part of the South of Europe, or the West Indies. Several striking cases of entire relief

[13] Anson Jones, *Memoranda and Official Correspondence Relating to the Republic of Texas, Its History and Annexation*, 11.

[14] Rev. Chester Newell, *A History of the Revolution in Texas*, preface.

> from these diseases are stated by persons of the highest intelligence and character.
>
> One of these is a gentleman, whose name as a patriot and statesman, holds a distinguished place in the history of Texas. He states that when he left his former residence in the United States, his frame was wasted to a skeleton, his strength was gone, and he was regarded by his friends as in the last stages of consumption. . . . but now, in the enjoyment of vigorous health, [he] exercises a powerful influence over the councils of his adopted country. . . . .
>
> Numerous other instances are related by the subjects of the diseases themselves or their immediate relatives, who, from pining and despairing weakness, accompanied with bleeding of the lungs, now enjoy a health apparently as sound and vigorous as any others.[15]

Even before 1840, some parts of Texas were in modest use by health-seekers; Sam Maverick, for instance, a victim of malaria when he arrived at Velasco in 1835, was advised by his friends to go to San Antonio, which was considered "more healthful" than the coastal towns. And William Bollaert, a perceptive English traveler, observed in 1843: "In the western [portion] and towards the mountain country, chills and fever are not known, and those who have been debilitated by it go to the West 'in search of health,' and a residence in San Antonio for a short time re-establishes them."[16] Thus it occurred that parts of Texas gradually came to be included within the framework of the western health frontier.

While the relations between Texas and Mexico remained unstable between 1836 and 1846, prewar contacts along the New Mexican border by other Americans proceeded on a rather peaceful basis, and made possible the continued flow of invalids into western regions. Indeed, in the years after 1840 hardly a wagon

15 Lawrence, *Texas in 1840: Emigrant's Guide to the New Republic*, 103.

16 Rena Maverick Green (ed.), *Samuel Maverick, Texan: 1803–1870*, 20; *William Bollaert's Texas*, 200. Bollaert, an accomplished naturalist, ethnologist, and geographer, not only traveled but also lived in the state.

train leaving for Santa Fe, or a hunting party departing for the Rockies, failed to include one or more of these pale-faced hulks, and their presence became so commonplace that their names appear almost matter-of-factly among the lists of travelers.[17]

Most representative of the pre–Mexican War prairie and mountain health travelers, and one who helped to publicize the climatic attractions of the West, was Matthew C. Field, thespian, bard, scribe, and consumptive. Field actually made two trips to the frontier for his health, one in 1839 to Santa Fe and another in 1843 into the Rocky Mountains. Upon his return from the first of these journeys, he was employed by the New Orleans *Picayune* as an assistant editor and feature writer, and between 1839 and 1841 he contributed a series of articles to the paper based on his western experiences, many of which were subsequently plagiarized and reprinted in journals across the nation. Among those directly influenced by his popular literary efforts was none other than his employer, George Wilkins Kendall, invalid Texan–Santa Fe tramp in 1841.[18]

Another series of articles equally popular followed the second of his jaunts, this one being made in the company of at least two other phthisics—William L. Sublette who led the hunting party into the mountains and Joseph Ogle from Illinois who "sought the mountains for health." That Field and his companions benefited from their exposure to the rarefied mountain air is clearly disclosed in this ringing excerpt of a letter published in the *Picayune* on November 7, 1843, shortly before his return:

> I seize the chance however to assure you of our full safety . . . and fine and flourishing condition of health. I will prove to you personally, your readers severally, panacea concoctors collectively

[17] See for example James Josiah Webb, *Adventures in the Santa Fe Trade 1844–47*, as reprinted in Ralph P. Bieber (ed.), *The Southwest Historical Series*, I, 47; and Matthew C. Field, *Prairie and Mountain Sketches, xxxi.*

[18] Matthew C. Field, *Matt Field on the Santa Fe Trail, xxv-xxvi;* Kendall also acknowledged the influence of Josiah Gregg in his decision to travel west for his health. *Texan Santa Fe Expedition, xxx,* 4.

> and all the doctors unequivocally, when I get home, that consumptives must no more "sparkle, exhale" and go to Havana, but jump into dresses of deerskin, and trot off to the mountains. We are the fattest, greasiest set of truant rogues your liveliest imagination can call up to view. . . . If you can get any of your Mesmerizers to give a clairvoyant view of our caravan and cavalcade, for the love of all that is grotesque and curious, drop off into magnetic somnolency and just take a look at us, do![19]

Hard on Matt Field's heels in the early 1840's came a surge of emigration along the overland routes to Oregon and California. Although these lands held a powerful appeal for Americans by that time, it took a special brand of courage and a peculiar set of conditions to cause men to detach themselves from friends and hard-won Valley lands. Untold dangers lurked along every mile of the vast stretches of the Oregon Trail, but apparently the unknown hazards were less to be feared by 1840 than the known threats of disease and death in the Mississippi Basin.

The first serious impetus to colonize Oregon was provided by Rev. Jason Lee. Having spent a number of years in that territory as a Methodist missionary, he returned to the states in 1838 and, in a series of recruiting and fund-raising lectures, told such encouraging stories of rich soils and healthy climate that a great deal of interest was generated in that remote Pacific country.[20]

His descriptions of Oregon's unqualified salubrity were, however, somewhat exaggerated; in fact, from the accounts of earlier travelers to that country, it appears that the climate of the region enjoyed at best a rather mixed reputation. Ross Cox, a visitor at Astoria in 1812, remarked that the climate was generally healthy, but Rev. Samuel Parker, an explorer in Oregon in 1835, recorded that about seven-eighths of the Indians in the region below the falls of the Columbia River had perished from fever and ague

[19] Field, *Prairie and Mountain Sketches, xxiv, xxxiv,* 118, 205.

[20] LeRoy R. Hafen and Ann W. Hafen (eds.), *To the Rockies and Oregon 1839–1842,* in *The Far West and Rockies Historical Series, 1820–1875,* III, 19–20, 144.

since 1829. Rev. Joseph Williams, another Methodist missionary who journeyed to Oregon in 1841, reported that the beautiful plains in the Willamette valley also were "somewhat sickly."[21] And as a general rule, all agreed that the best health was to be found at some distance above the falls of the various rivers in the Columbia River Basin. Thus, Lee's remarks appear to have been filled more with enthusiasm than with reality, but even then it is quite likely that conditions of health in the Oregon country were superior to those found in the interior valley.

Most interesting of those who responded favorably to Lee's thrilling lectures was Thomas J. Farnham, a man destined to cast his influence (much of it adverse) on the settlement of both Oregon and California. Farnham, "an invalid, hopelessly gone with consumption it was thought," left a promising legal career in New York around 1837 and moved to the West in search of a climate cure for his distresses.[22] Life among the trappers in the Rocky Mountains proved so beneficial that after only a short residence he recovered his health and was able to resume his practice in Peoria, Illinois. It was in that city in 1838 that Jason Lee stirred Farnham with an intense "patriotic fervor" to wrest control of the Oregon lands from the powerful British Hudson's Bay Company.

"On the 21st of May, 1839," Farnham wrote in his journals, "the author and sixteen others arrived in the town of Independence, Missouri. . . . Some of our number sought health in the wilderness—others sought the wilderness for its own sake—and others sought a residence [in] the valley of the Columbia." The party, nineteen in number by the time of its departure, consti-

[21] Ross Cox, *The Columbia River* (ed. by Edgar I. and Jane R. Stewart), 233, 252, 257; Rev. Samuel Parker, *Journal of an Exploring Tour Beyond the Rocky Mountains,* 191; Hafen and Hafen, *To the Rockies and Oregon,* in *The Far West and Rockies Historical Series,* III, 255.

[22] Bidwell, *Echoes of the Past,* 16.

tuted the first of such groups to embark on the overland trails to the then disputed Oregon territory.

Dissension, hardship, and discouragement reduced the Farnham-led Peoria party to three members before its October arrival at Fort Walla Walla. A bone-weary Farnham was sorely disappointed at what he saw there. For a country that had been represented as fruitful and beautiful, he wrote rather dejectedly, "I am obliged to deny so foul an imputation upon the fair fame of dame Nature. It is an ugly desert; designed to be such, made such, and is such." Although his enthusiasm was dulled by his observations, he nonetheless made one feeble, abortive effort to persuade the United States to take over the protection of the territory with a petition, signed by some seventy settlers, in which Oregon was represented as "one of the most favored portions of the globe." This failing, he soon departed by sea for the states leaving behind a country only one-third of which he had found to possess "a pure and healthy air."[23]

Of the later invalids who resorted to an Oregon excursion, Francis Parkman, whose *The Oregon Trail* is a classic on that portion of the West, made the trip in 1846. A major reason why he made the journey was an attempt to improve his declining health. In this he failed, but it is highly improbable that any climatic change would have benefited the palsied nervous debilitations which made his life a continual nightmare. Additionally, J. Quinn Thornton, along with his wife who also was in ill health, went to Oregon in 1848 hoping to restore the "inestimable blessing [they] had lost," and apparently both succeeded.[24] The reports of these men, though only moderately favorable to the

[23] Thomas J. Farnham, *Travels in the Great Western Prairies,* in Thwaites' *Early Western Travels,* XXVIII, 35, 84–86, 347.

[24] Dumas Malone (ed.), *Dictionary of American Biography,* XIV, 247; J. Quinn Thornton, *Oregon and California in 1848,* I, 13; a good description of the climate in Oregon may be found on the pages following 357.

health-seeker, did nothing to discredit the acknowledged fertility of great portions of the land in the Oregon territory, and thousands presently entered the region as homesteaders. But as a health resort, the country offered only a fraction of the appeal which many cismontane locations had achieved by the forties. This was not to be true for parts of California.

On his return route from Oregon in 1840, Thomas Farnham landed in strife-torn Mexican California, then dominated by Anastasio Bustamante's Centralists, and at Monterey viewed first-hand the mistreatment of a group of Americans accused of supporting Liberalist activities there. The episode formed the basis of his discouraging reports on that portion of the Pacific coast, reports which subsequently had a near-paralyzing effect on John Bidwell's attempt to organize the first party of overland Californians in 1841.

The fire of enthusiasm which Antoine Robidoux had kindled among Missourians in 1840 smouldered rapidly into ashes of apathy following the circulation of Farnham's spirit-dampening letters in frontier newspapers. Of the five hundred men who signed the initial pledge to move to California in that year, only Bidwell thereafter remained firm in his determination to do so. Throughout the winter months that followed, a financially embarrassed and intensely dejected Bidwell could reactivate little interest in the proposed venture until an invalid from Illinois, George Henshaw, agreed to provide him with a much-needed yoke of oxen in exchange for the right to accompany him across the prairies, a transaction which to Bidwell seemed "almost providential."[25] From this partnership the number of interested people eventually grew to seventy men, women, and children, and in the spring of 1841 this modest party set out for Robidoux's "perfect paradise."

Bidwell's journal comments are uncommonly generous on the

[25] Bidwell, *Echoes of the Past,* 21.

healthfulness of California, and though he does not mention their names, apparently several health-seekers were among his party, all of whom had recovered by the time their destination was reached. The following excerpts are indicative of Bidwell's reflections:

> The country is acknowledged by all to be extremely healthy, there is no disease common to the country, the fever and ague are seldom known. . . . Let me here remark that those of the Company who came here for their health, were all successful. A young man by name of Walton, who, when he set out was of a death like appearance—having been afflicted with dropsy or consumption, landed in perfect health. . . . To all of my acquaintances and friends, who may be in bad health I would recommend a trip to California. All, whom I have heard speak of the climate as regarded their health, say its effects have been salutary.[26]

Although Bidwell's party was the first to cross the prairies to sunny California, the real credit for opening the famed, and much used, California Trail went to the Stevens party in 1844. Sometimes referred to as the Townsend or Murphy party after two of its more prominent members, this group not only discovered the Trail but also brought back its exact location to other prospective emigrants.

The Murphy of this party was Martin Murphy, Sr., of St. Joseph, Missouri. An Irish immigrant to Canada in 1820, Murphy moved his family in 1840 "across the then western wilds" to Missouri hoping to find deep, fertile soils. These he found, but health he did not find. Within a short time all of the settlers in his area were attacked by deadly malaria, and some members of his own family died from the disease. It was then that Father Hookins, a Roman Catholic missionary, visited the settlement and found Murphy "mourning over [the] loss of loved ones and full of anxiety as to the fate of the others who were sick." Drawing upon descriptions obtained from church brothers who had served in

[26] John Bidwell, [*Journal of a Trip to California in 1841*], 27, 29, 32.

California missions, the priest told the bereaved family of the "glorious climate and fertile soil" in that remote region of the West. On the strength of Father Hookins' testimony, the elder Murphy decided to remove his family from the "puker's purgatory" and to seek a new life in the "cougher's paradise."

These pilgrims, along with the rest of the Stevens party, endured unusual hardships during their eight months' (May, 1844, to January, 1845) journey over plains, deserts, and mountains, but their sufferings were not in vain. California was, indeed, as it had been described; "their hopes had ended in fruition."[27] Bayard Taylor, a traveling reporter for Horace Greeley's New York *Tribune,* visited the Murphys in 1849 and described the valley in which their ranch was located as luxuriantly fertile with a soft, balmy atmosphere which he "may have seen equaled but never surpassed."[28]

While the call to distant Oregon and California grew stronger every day, the Mormons became the first large group to make a successful settlement in the central Rocky Mountains. Put to flight by the evil winds of religious conflict, these Brigham Young–led "saints" left their Nauvoo homes in 1846 and fled to a new sanctuary in the Great Salt Flats of Utah. Some of their number combined a quest for religious freedom with a search for personal health. William Chandless, an English traveler who followed one of the Mormon parties to Salt Lake, told of engaging the services of a young physician who "had regularly studied and practiced in Philadelphia, and had rather come on the plains as a cure for pulmonary weakness than from any special zeal for Mormonism." And in a footnote he demonstrated how widespread the health legend had become:

> Whatever be the cause, it is found as a fact that those suffering from pulmonary diseases in the Eastern States are much bene-

[27] Moses Schallenberger, *The Opening of the California Trail,* 24, 48–49, 83.
[28] Bayard Taylor, *Eldorado: Or Adventures in the Path of Empire,* 96.

fited by traveling West; and the converse is found true to a great extent. This I have heard both in Illinois and Minnesota.[29]

Thus did the Mormons, last of the pre–Mexican War groups to "invade" Mexican territory, give impetus to the expansion of the health frontier.

Health-seekers were found even among the United States army units which marched southwestward in 1846 to fight the Mexican War. Susan Magoffin, delicate bride of a New Mexican trader and passenger in a group that followed the Kearny expedition to Santa Fe, wrote in her diary that she "never should have consented to take the trip on the plains had it not been with the view and a hope that it would prove beneficial" to her health. Josiah Gregg, the inveterate prairie traveler whose health had again failed during the period of his medical studies, joined a group of Arkansas volunteers en route to Texas and Mexico "as well for my health as to endeavor . . . to be of any service to my country." And Lieutenant J. W. Abert, an officer under the command of General Kearny, almost missed the war when fever and ague struck him down near Bent's Fort, but he arose from a convalescent's bed in August, 1846, and made long, forced marches in the dry Southwest atmosphere with his men because he "knew that this exercise would be of great . . . benefit" to a constitution which had not yet entirely recovered from the severe shock it had sustained a month earlier.[30]

Military reports arising from the war greatly reinforced and substantially verified the previously established claims to healthfulness of many of the regions through which the various army units passed. Captain George W. Hughes, topographical engineer with the Arkansas volunteers, recorded that San Antonio was a "healthy and beautiful town," that the vicinity around it

29 William Chandless, *A Visit to Salt Lake*, 59–60, 60 n.

30 Magoffin, *Down the Santa Fe Trail*, 63–65; *Diary and Letters of Josiah Gregg*, I, 197, 200; J. W. Abert, *Report . . . of His Examination of New Mexico, in the Years 1846–47*, 3, 92.

also was "said to be very healthy," and that there was "apparently no cause for disease." Dr. Frederick Adolphus Wislizenus, a physician connected with Colonel Doniphan's expedition, wrote glowingly of the "temperate, constant, and healthy" climate of New Mexico, and observed that "disease seems to be very little known" except for minor inflammations during the winter months. Lieutenant William H. Emory, who accompanied General Kearny's overland strike into California, found the climate in the southern coastal regions almost unsurpassed in salubrity, and recorded: "With the exception of a very few cases of ague and fever of a mild type, sickness is unknown."[31] Emory's estimates were generous, and for southern California were accurate, but they were not to prove characteristic for all of the state—a fact to which many a forty-niner would presently attest.

A multitude of ambitious Argonauts and adventurers put reports like that of the young army lieutenant to a rigid test in the first few years after the Mexican War, and in doing so they unwittingly provided invaluable information on the extent of the health frontier in California. Months before the gold rush began, J. Q. Thornton had cautioned prospective immigrants that the fertile valleys of the San Joaquin and Sacramento rivers were "somewhat sickly during the months of September, October, and November when . . . vegetation decomposes and fills the air with malaria."[32] Such a declaration should have been a familiar omen to residents of the eastern states and particularly of the Mississippi Valley, but the warning seems to have deterred them not at all. Many were destined to learn the bitter truth of Thornton's admonition.

The mining camps became virtual death traps in the early

[31] George W. Hughes, *Memoir: Descriptive of the March of a Division of the United States Army, under the Command of Brigadier General John E. Wool*, 9–11; Frederick Adolphus Wislizenus, *Memoir of a Tour to Northern Mexico Connected with Col. Doniphan's Expedition in 1846 and 1847*, 25; William Hemsley Emory, *Lieutenant Emory Reports*, 195–96.

[32] Thornton, *Oregon and California in 1848*, II, 83.

years, largely on account of inadequate food, improper shelter, and damp working conditions. There was in addition the serious problem of acclimation. "There was much sickness among the miners," one observer wrote, "especially those who had recently arrived in the country."[33] Another recorded that scores of pale, emaciated frames, "broken down by Agues and diarrhoeas," were arriving daily in San Francisco from the Sacramento and its tributaries. And he concluded:

> At least one third of the miners suffered more or less from these diseases, and numbers of men who had landed only a few months before, in the fulness of hale and lusty manhood, were walking about nearly as shrunken and bloodless as the corpses they would soon become.[34]

Overall, only the southern portions of the state afforded a disease-free environment; this fact is clearly evidenced in the following summary made by an invalid in 1862:

> Many parts of the state, especially those near the coast, are very healthy. Indeed, I do not think that in any part of the world is nature more favorable to long life than in California from Sonoma to Santa Barbara, within thirty miles of the ocean. . . . In the low land of the Sacramento and Colorado basins, . . . the health of the inhabitants is not so good. In many of the mining towns . . . fever and ague are common. That disease prevails also in the moist lands along the Sacramento and San Joaquin Rivers. . . . Rheumatism is very common in the mines, and neuralgia throughout the state. . . . Diseases of the eyes are common here. . . . The dense fogs which visit the coast render the climate unfavorable to persons afflicted with consumption; while I presume a residence in the mountains high above the sea, would be very likely to cure that disease, at least in its early stages.[35]

Since it was customary for health-seekers to seize any oppor-

[33] Alonzo Delano, *Life on the Plains and Among the Diggings,* 256; John Steele, *In Camp and Cabin,* 151.

[34] B. Taylor, *Eldorado,* 154.

[35] John S. Hittell, *The Resources of California,* 367–68.

tunity to cross the plains and prairies, the presence of a small number of them among parties bound for the gold fields was hardly precedent-shattering. Indeed the prospect of finding wealth as well as health made California doubly alluring. Benjamin Butler Harris, a resident on the East Texas fringe of the Mississippi Basin, joined one of the earliest Argonaut trains to depart from Texas for California. He took his legal practice and a bad liver farther west because he was convinced that the "Brazos fever," a form of malaria which "like a juggling devil assaulted [him] front and rear and hung like an incubus upon [his] constitution," would do him in if he remained. Alonzo Delano, whose body "had suffered sad inroads by disease incident to western climate," left Ohio with a California-bound wagon train in April, 1849, besieged with a fever of the body as well as a "fever of mind for gold."[36] Both of these men recovered and prospered after reaching the Pacific Coast.

Shortly after southern California became identified with the western health frontier, encouraging reports began to circulate on the climatic attractions of the Arizona territory, last of the regions of the Southwest to be included within the framework of the resort area. Rufus B. Sage, an invalid who traveled in the western country in 1845, visited the Colorado and Gila country and wrote quite convincingly of its healthfulness.

> There are many sweet spots in the vicinity of both these streams, well deserving the name of earthly Edens. Man here might fare sumptuously, with one continued feast spread before him by the spontaneous products of the earth, and revel in perennial spring or luxurate amid unfading summer. . . . The entire [region] possesses a uniformly salubrious and healthful atmosphere. Sickness, so far as my knowledge extends, is rarely known.[37]

[36] Benjamin Butler Harris, *The Gila Trail: The Texas Argonauts and the California Gold Rush,* 7; Delano, *Life on the Plains and Among the Diggings,* 13–14.
[37] Rufus B. Sage, *Scenes in the Rocky Mountains,* 237.

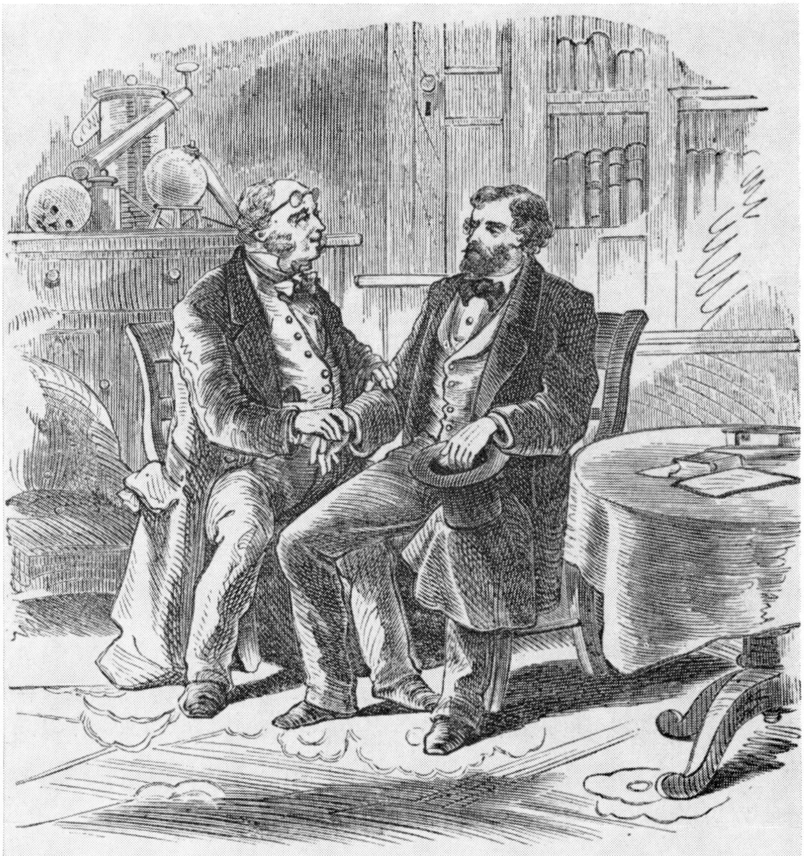

"GO WEST, YOUNG MAN; GO WEST!"

Whether in the first or last stages of illnesses and sometimes no matter what the diagnosis, patients were frequently advised to "go west" for "climate cure."

From John Hanson Beadle's *The Undeveloped West; or Five Years in the Territories,* courtesy Denver Public Library Western Collection

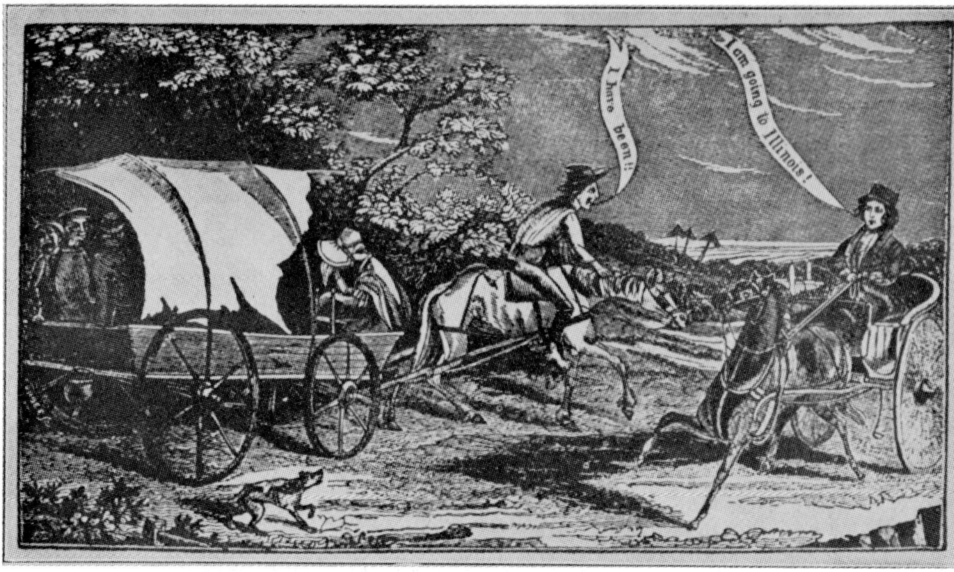

After a year's residence in the "highly extolled country of Illinois" this traveler returned with "a *broken* down wagon—a *broken* winded horse!—a *broken* hearted wife!—a *broken* legged dog;—and . . . the irreparable *broken* constitution" of three "*Fever and Ague* sons."

From Wilkey's *Western Emigration* (1839)

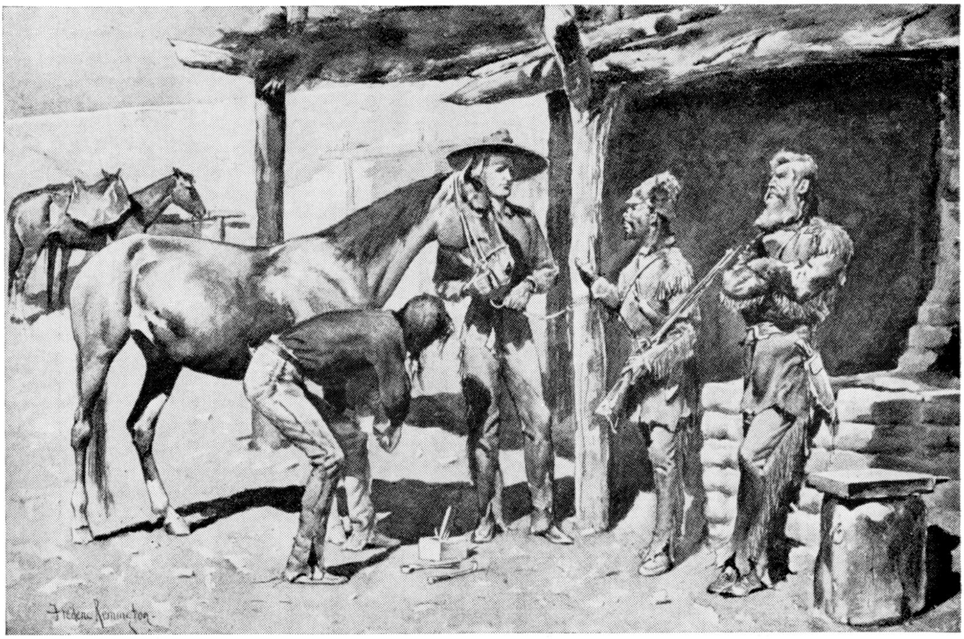

Francis Parkman at Fort Laramie in 1846 as depicted by Frederic Remington. The future historian of the Oregon Trail wrote his father, "This country is remarkably healthy. . . . I am in very excellent health."

From the de luxe 1892 edition of Parkman's *The Oregon Trail*

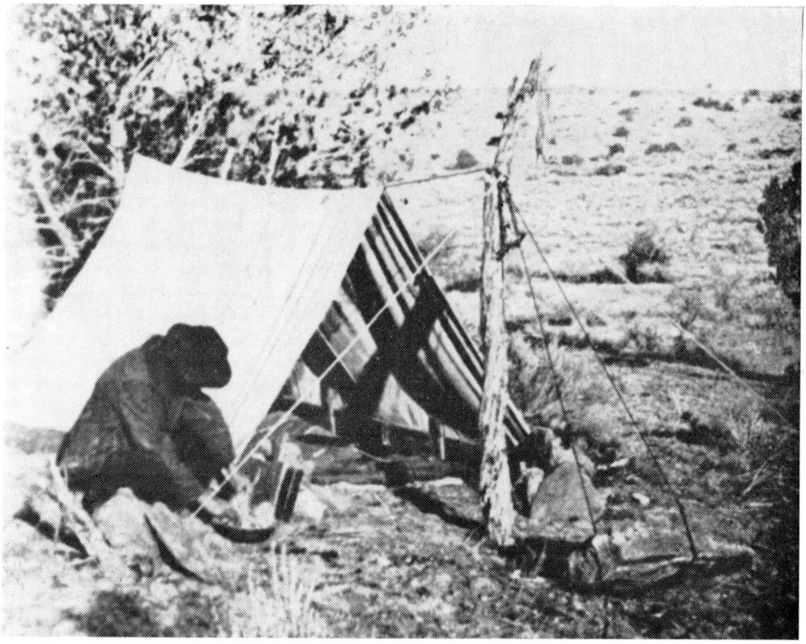

This health-seeker, who has pitched his pup tent in arid country, needs only load his pack on his four-legged companion to become a "burro tourist."

From Sharlot M. Hall's "Burden of the Southwest," *Out West*, Vol. XXVIII (January, 1908)

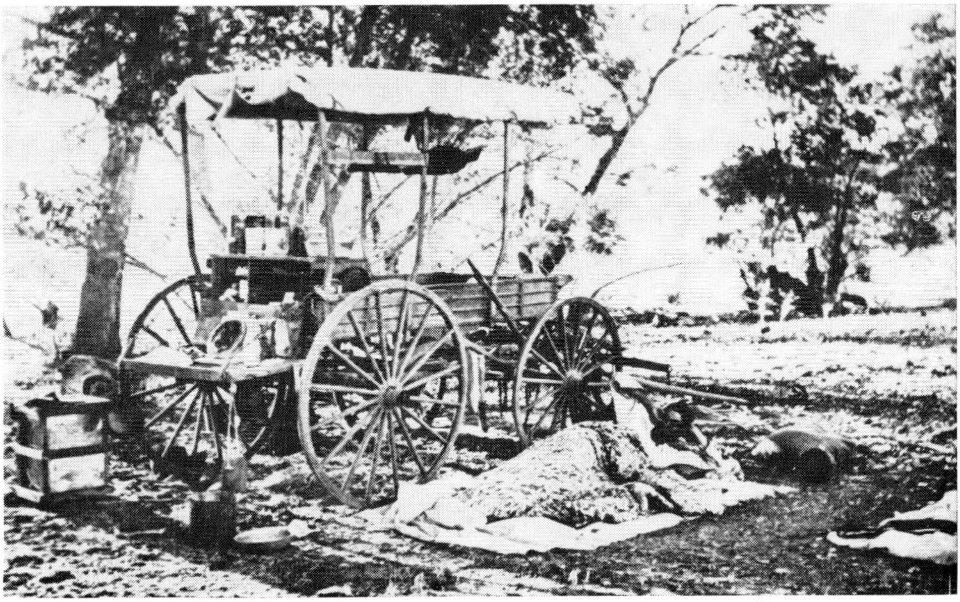

Sunshine, fresh air, and simple diet was the road to health for many tuberculars living a wagon-home existence in austere and isolated locales.

From Sharlot M. Hall's "Burden of the Southwest," *Out West*, Vol. XXVIII (January, 1908)

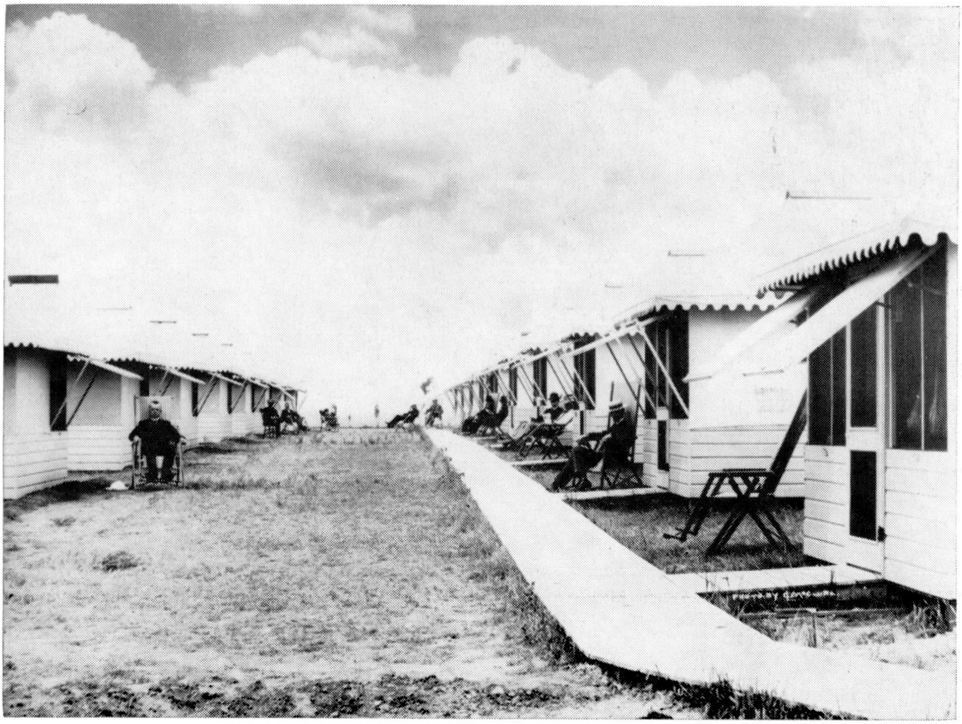

Patients relaxing in the sunshine and fresh air at Agnes Memorial Sanatorium, Denver.

Photograph by L. C. McClure, courtesy Denver Library Western Collection

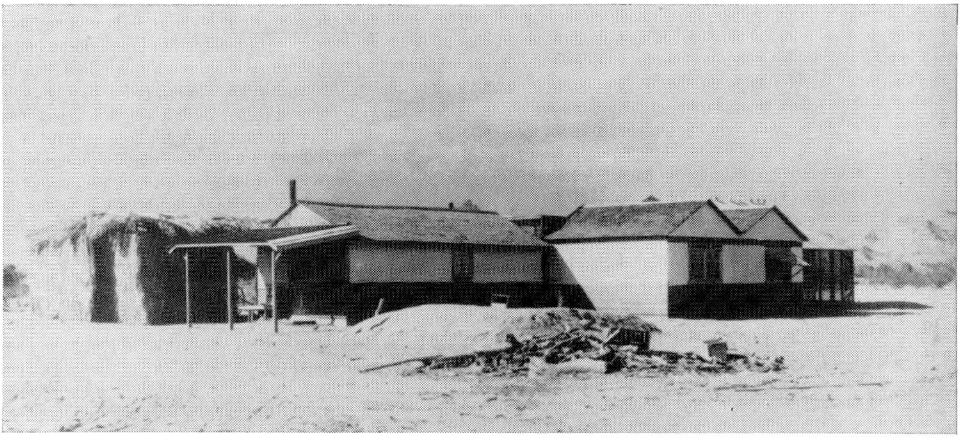

A "lunger's" oasis, a camp on the desert near Phoenix, Arizona.

Courtesy Arizona Historical Foundation, Phoenix

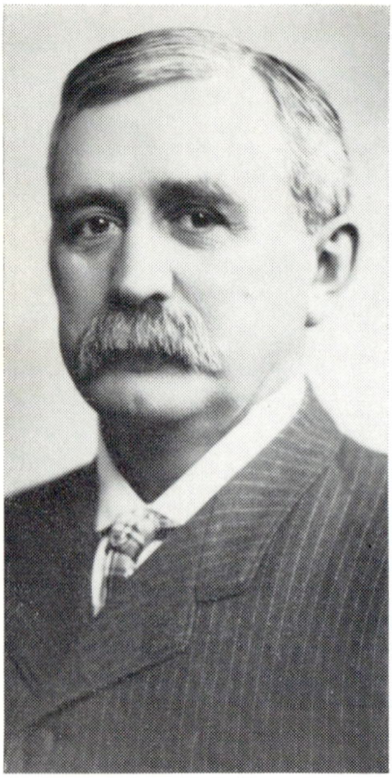

Dr. Charles Denison

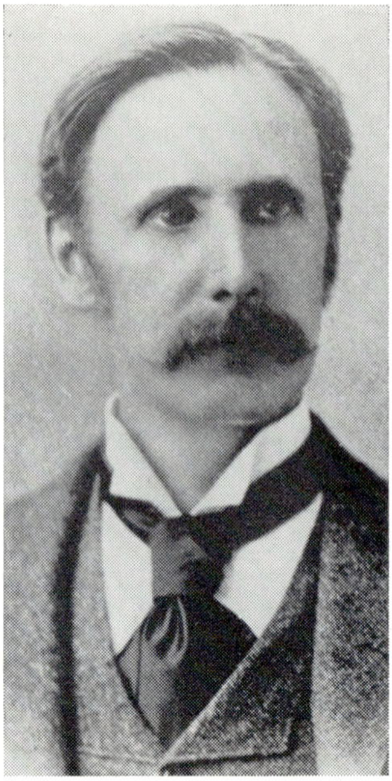

Dr. Samuel Edwin Solly

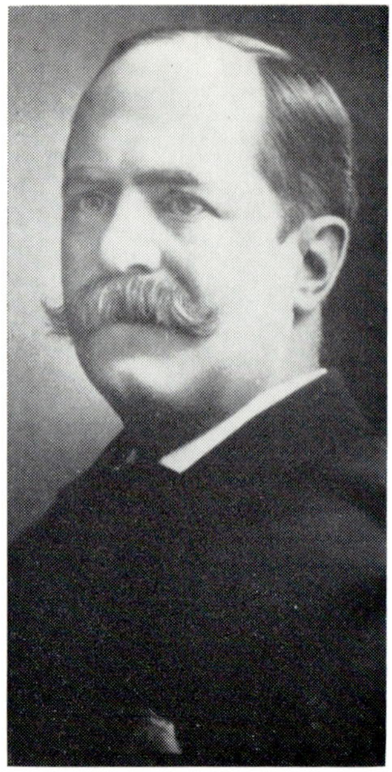

Dr. Samuel A. Fisk

This Colorado triumvirate of the American Climatological Association, themselves tuberculars, played dramatic roles in attempting to develop a science of climate and its effects on respiratory diseases.

All photographs courtesy Denver Public Library Western Collection

The extreme aridity of Arizona and its infestation with hostile red men were facts well known to most Americans, and for these reasons the lands of the two southwestern rivers were none too enticing despite Sage's encouraging summary. American ownership of the region after the Mexican War and increasing migrations across it to California, however, gave Arizona a new importance; the expediency of establishing permanent roads and communication linkages across that portion of the Southwest became paramount considerations.

From the records of the various surveying teams that explored the country, it is possible to fix the origin of some of the later reports on Arizona's salubrity. Edward Fitzgerald Beale, commissioned in 1857 to lay out a wagon road from Fort Defiance (Arizona) to the Colorado River, wrote to the War Department:

> In the journey of the year, during which I have been engaged in this work, I have not lost a man, nor was there the slightest case of sickness in camp; the medicine chest proved only an encumbrance. My surgeon having left me, at the commencement of the journey, I did not employ, nor did I have need of one on the entire road.[38]

And Major J. C. Woods, who helped to pioneer an overland mail route from San Antonio to San Diego, sent the following report to the Post Office Department in 1857:

> I never had a case of sickness among either men or passengers during my whole trip, excepting a little annoyance from an over indulgence in fruit in the valley of the Rio Grande. The salubrious air must be conducive to health.[39]

The faith men developed in the efficacy of western climates seemed more than justified in the light of an increasing number of invalids who benefited from a tour across the plains and mountains. There was, however, ample evidence extant to the careful

[38] Edward F. Beale, *Wagon Road from Fort Defiance to the Colorado River*, 4.
[39] *Texas Almanac for 1859*, 145.

observer which proved unquestionably that prairie therapeutics, though of undoubted value, were far from the panacea they were purported to be. Albert D. Richardson noted, for instance, that the average migrant who traveled westward was thankful when he reached the Rocky Mountains, "for the road by which he came had been passed over successively by Oregon pioneers, soldiers, Mormons, and California emigrants, and was dotted with graves thicker than milestones."[40] Franklin Langworthy, an overland traveler to the gold fields in 1850, in like manner wrote:

> Graves are so numerous, that to notice them all, would make my narrative tedious . . . there has been more than one thousand emigrants buried upon the road to California, during last year and the present season . . . the principal part have fallen victim of that fearful scourge, the cholera. In some instances, every person belonging to a wagon has died of the pestilence.[41]

As further evidence of the mixed effect of western climate, the following citations are presented as they were recorded in some of the travelers' accounts of the day:

> News soon arrived of the . . . death of the sick man, Bishop, who was bound for the Rocky Mountains for his health.
>
> Last night a Mr. Phelps, who had left his home to try the health restoring climate of the Rocky Mountains, died. Being in the last stage of consumption, he had hoped that the pure air of the prairies might ameliorate his diseases.
>
> Col. Owen's Company which got before us this morning, were just starting after performing the last office to the dead body of a Mexican. He had consumption. Poor man, 'twas but yesterday that we sent him some soup from our camp. . . .
>
> A short distance from our place of encampment, I observed a newly made grave, . . . and in examining the wooden head board, I found it to be the last resting place of George W. Tindal, . . . who had died of consumption.

[40] Richardson, *Our New States and Territories*, 12.
[41] Franklin Langworthy, *Scenery of the Plains, Mountains and Mines*, 46.

> This evening Mr. S. H. Wilson of Dodgeville died in camp. He had for some [time] had poor health and started on this journey with the hope of recovering his health. But here his journey ended.[42]

Thus it seems certain that those who helped to promote a legend of perfect health in the West all too frequently ignored the grim realities of numerous poorly marked graves and many casually recorded deaths. Like the clairvoyant physician, the West's reputation was built only upon successes; the restoration of a single invalid was enough to obscure a hundred failures. Unlike the medical fraud, however, western climate achieved well-deserved respect not only because a large number of men benefited from it but also because it offered a welcomed contrast to residents of the disease-ridden Mississippi Valley.

Promotion of the health legend proceeded rapidly after the Mexican War. Men with national, even international, reputations endorsed climatic therapy and made it easier for others to accept the premise of a disease-free and health-restoring environment in the western prairies and mountains. George Frederick Ruxton, world-famed adventurer and widely read author, resorted to his "beloved Rockies" in 1848 in an effort to find renewed health and was obliged to sell his royalty rights to *Life in the Far West* in order to make the trip. He later acknowledged having known more than a hundred tuberculars who had been virtually resurrected from the grave by a winter's residence in the southern Rocky Mountains.[43] And Frederick Law Olmsted, well-known author and pre–Civil War traveler among the southern states, took along his consumptive brother, Dr. John H. Olmsted, when he made his famous saddle trip through Texas in

[42] Edward Evans Parrish, *Crossing the Plains in 1844*, 84; Abert, *Report . . . of His Examination*, 84; Magoffin, *Down the Santa Fe Trail*, 38; Delano, *Life on the Plains and Among the Diggings*, 68; Edward Dunsha Steele, *Edward Dunsha Steele*, 1829–1865, 73. Citations in order of reference sequence above.

[43] George Frederick Ruxton, *Ruxton of the Rockies* (ed. by LeRoy R. Hafen), 269.

1856–57. The Olmsteds' reactions to the sanative effects of such a trip are worth noting because of the encouragement they offered to other prospective emigrants:

> . . . to a pulmonary invalid, who can throw off cares, and who has any recuperative elasticity in him, I can recommend nothing more heartily than a winter's ride . . . upon the Texan prairies. For many a case of incipient phthisis, such a course of six months of leisurely prairie-life, . . . would, for many a man, now hacking away at his young tubercules in hot rooms, . . . double not only the length but the enjoyable value of life, and at not greater outlay than the sum of his medical bills.[44]

Noninvalids joined them in singing praises to western climates. Hoarce Greeley was almost poetic in describing the attractiveness of the Rocky Mountains:

> . . . the Rocky Mountains, with their grand, aromatic forests, their grassey glades, their frequent springs, and dancing streams of the brightest, sweetest water, their pure, elastic atmosphere, and their unequalled game and fish, are destined to be a favorite resort and home of civilized man. I never visited a region where physical life could be more surely prolonged or fully enjoyed.[45]

Others were equally praiseworthy in their descriptions of the salubrious West. "You may talk of your sound sleepers," Douglas Brewerton wrote after a visit to New Mexico in 1854, "on featherbeds in well-ceiled chambers, you city bred people, who fancy you are enjoying robust health." But, he retorted:

> What do you know of "Nature's sweet restorer?" Why, I would not give one hour of that dreamless repose beneath the open sky, with the star-lit heavens above, and the pure night winds as they come surging over the dew-laden grasses . . . for all your feverish visions, born of indigestion and an impure atmosphere.[46]

[44] Frederick Law Olmstead, *A Journey Through Texas,* 380–81.

[45] Horace Greeley, *An Overlord Journey,* 136.

[46] G. Douglas Brewerton, "Incidents of Travel in New Mexico," *Harper's New Monthly Magazine,* Vol. VIII (April, 1854), 582.

And finally, W. W. H. Davis in 1857 recorded in a similar vein:

> Out on these great plains a person experiences different feelings than when confined within cities. . . . He appears to breathe deeper, and to increase in stature; the sky seems to be bluer and cleaner, the air purer, and the sun to shine more brightly . . . in beholding Nature's works. . . . A man . . . cannot fail to be made better and wiser by a trip across the prairies. . . . Health [in New Mexico] seems to be the natural condition of man instead of disease, and a larger number of persons live to a great old age than in any other part of our country, and before they die some assume almost the appearance of Egyptian mummies.[47]

The increasing amount of promotional rhetoric which appeared throughout the 1850's is unmistakable proof that the health legend had reached a significant degree of maturity and acceptance. Additionally, by 1860 the locations of the most favorable areas had become common knowledge to most Americans and to many Europeans. The broad outlines of the health frontier were known to include the middle and southern Rockies from Denver to Santa Fe and Albuquerque, and the southwestern prairies, plains, and deserts from San Antonio to San Diego and Santa Barbara. To these, portions of the Columbia River Basin could be added, but because of their inaccessibility, Oregon lands remained only loosely associated with what was predominantly a southwestern health frontier.

But if by 1860 the framework of this frontier had been completed, a man-made barrier—the Civil War—postponed temporarily its inevitable exploitation.

[47] W. W. H. Davis, *El Gringo: New Mexico and Her People,* 24, 295.

V. *Early Promotion and Settlement of the Health Frontier, 1865-90*

For most Americans the period of the Civil War was one of intensified activity and desperate fighting, but for the health-seeker it was an agonizing hiatus in the development of plains and mountain resort areas. The western surge ended rather abruptly in 1861, and few opportunities thereafter were available for diseased Valley residents to travel to the more healthful regions until peace was restored. With war's end, an avalanche of invalids, made impatient by four long years of waiting, spilled into the trans-Mississippi West and participated throughout the remainder of the century in settling the nation's last frontier.

During the war years, a few bits of encouraging information in widely scattered sources continued to circulate in the eastern states, but these had little effect on the public other than to remind it of the atmospheric blessings which would greet the resumption of western traffic. Miners' guidebooks were particularly tantalizing in their descriptions not only of material resources of newly discovered Rocky Mountain gold fields but also of the climatic attractions of the various regions. "Thus far," one account read, "the climate has proved to be very healthy." "No sickness," another detailed, "occurred at the mines last year, and old mountaineers say they know nothing about sickness." Still another stated that "the record of mortality, since the first settlement of the country [Colorado], exhibits a remarkable degree of healthfulness, the air is at all times pure, bracing, and invigorating, and entirely free from the malaria generally encountered in newly settled regions."[1]

Easily the most enticing of the wartime reports was written by Maurice O'Connor Morris in 1864:

> When I first arrived [at Denver, Colorado], I was greatly struck by the different appearances of the faces here from the eastern visages I had just left. There, dyspepsia or the affects of fever and ague, or consumption, were too plainly written to be ignored by any passerby, on a very large percentage of the population; here I see nothing but health visible.[2]

Along with some excellent and encouraging rhetoric, Morris revealed rather conspicuously that nothing had occurred during the war years to mitigate the distressing, insalubrious environment of the Mississippi Basin. Conditions were largely as they had always been—deplorable—and were to remain so for an indefinite period. Proof of this fact was shown by Edward Tenney who recorded in 1880 that there was hardly a well woman in the whole of Illinois, and he further remarked, "Multitudes of people in the valley of the Mississippi are slowly dying within two days' ride of perfect health."[3]

Expediency and opportunity do not tell the complete story of the postwar surge to the frontier; as in previous periods of western development, the reports of travelers served only to increase knowledge of and to promote interest in the undeveloped regions. No portion of the health frontier, with the possible exception of southern California, received greater nationwide publicity after the Civil War than Colorado, and this at a time when crossing

[1] S. W. Burt and E. L. Berthoud, *The Rocky Mountain Gold Regions*, 24; *Miners' Hand-Book and Guide to Pike's Peak*, 18; William S. Rockwell, *Colorado: Its Mineral and Agricultural Resources*, 6.

[2] Maurice O'Connor Morris, *Rambles in the Rocky Mountains*, 88–89.

[3] Edward P. Tenney, *Colorado: New Homes in the West*, 41.

the plains was no easy task. Before railroads revolutionized transportation, early travelers could reach the Rocky Mountains aristocratically by stagecoach, democratically on foot, or respectably with a horse or oxteam. Most men traveled respectably either by necessity or for convenience, and such a journey required from thirty to sixty days, depending upon point of origin and weather along the route. After the Union Pacific crossed the plains, a traveler could reach the mountains luxuriously and rapidly, riding in day coaches or Pullman cars on a trip that took from two to four days. Whatever mode of travel was used, visiting scribes were thoroughly impressed with what they observed in the Centennial State and thereafter greatly influenced their readers with vivid descriptions of its stimulating environment.

Among the earliest of the postwar travelers was Samuel Bowles, who made a stage trip across the continent in 1865. He commented favorably on the health of several areas, but he reserved the highest praise for Colorado. He was so captivated by its invigorating atmosphere that he predicted it would one day become the Switzerland of America, an idea which was to be perpetuated by subsequent travelers. "When the Pacific Railroad is done," he prophesied, "our Switzerland will be at our very doors." And in a later publication he described Colorado as having

> over all an atmosphere so pure that the eye seems to take in all space, and so dry and exhilarating that life titillates at every avenue, and we mount as if on angel's wings. Here would seem to be the fountain of health; and among these hills and plains is surely to be many a summer resort for the invalid and the pleasure-seeker in the by no means distant future.[4]

Bayard Taylor, the California wanderer of an earlier period, visited Colorado the summer following Bowles's trek, and his reflections were almost identical with those of his predecessor.

[4] Samuel Bowles, *Across the Continent,* 31; Samuel Bowles, *The Switzerland of America,* 19.

He noticed very little sickness of any kind, found the people "remarkably healthy," and was told that diseases of the lungs were "almost always healed in this high and dry atmosphere." But, in what must have been one of the earliest warnings on the limitations of western climate, he cautioned his readers that here was, at the same time, less recuperative power once a person was attacked. He further warned that advanced cases of tuberculosis frequently terminated fatally. Despite these grim admonitions, Taylor predicted, in typical Bowles fashion, that Colorado would soon be recognized as "our Switzerland" and declared: "It will be a national blessing when this region is opened to general travel."[5]

For those who needed greater assurance than mere descriptive phraseology, such men as Albert D. Richardson, George W. Pine, and J. H. Beadle provided more direct evidence. Richardson, for example, testified in 1866:

> I have seen a lady ill with typhoid fever, and barely able to sit up, travel across the plains, and reach the end of an unintermitting stage journey of seven days and nights, with the roses restored to her cheek and vigor in her frame. I once knew a resident of Eastern Kansas, pronounced dying with consumption, who started on the long jaunt. Too weak to sit erect, he was placed upon a featherbed in an ox-wagon, sleeping in the open air every night; and when, after fifty days, he reached the Rocky Mountains, he was enjoying comfortable health.[6]

The following year, Richardson, en route again to the West, was himself prostrated at Fort Smith for weeks by typhoid fever, and though he recovered sufficiently to resume his journey, he wrote that the last vestiges of his illness were removed only after he had spent some time in the Rockies.[7]

George Pine combined rhetoric with evidence in his 1870 de-

[5] B. Taylor, *Colorado: A Summer Trip,* 58, 114, 166.
[6] Richardson, *Our New States and Territories,* 26.
[7] Richardson, *Beyond the Mississippi,* 218, 278.

scriptions of the climate of Colorado. In a summary which hardly seems original, he declared:

> . . . in this invigorating atmosphere lies the pleasure ground and health giving home of the nation. . . . An atmosphere so pure that the eye seems to take in all space, and so dry and exhilarating that life dances at every pore. You go about as on easy wings, light-hearted, having partaken freely at the fountain of pure health, . . . I saw some persons, supposed to be hopelessly consumptive, able only to travel in wagons, lying upon feather-beds, who, after crossing the plains and living in the mountains a while, recovered, so that they enjoyed a comfortable degree of health for years after. . . . Lung diseases, which in low country climates are so common and often so fatal, are almost surely cured in this high and arid atmosphere.[8]

Plagiarism or not, Pine's work was no less influential than the others, and he made it even more readable by occasionally adding a touch of the fantastic: "I was told that in some sections, it was so healthy that a man had to be killed to start a burying-ground."

J. H. Beadle's influence arose not so much from his descriptions of the Rocky Mountains as from his own recovery in the western climate. He was, in effect, the Josiah Gregg of the post–Civil War period. January, 1868, found him an invalid in Evansville, Indiana; a bronchial difficulty, produced by ten years of severe application to study and aggravated by a year of army life and by the "moist and enervating climate of Southern Indiana," had shackled him with "an ominous graveyard cough."[9]

After a desperate but futile search for a cure, he followed his physician's advice and "went west." In an effort to toughen himself for the task, Beadle began his journey as a pedestrian, and though he proceeded slowly, he became strong enough to walk thirty-five miles in a single day by the time he reached Iowa.

[8] George W. Pine, *Beyond the West*, 116–17.

[9] Beadle, *The Undeveloped West; or, Five Years in the Territories*, 33ff., 441.

This, he declared, was "not bad for an invalid," and he pronounced himself "ready for the plains."

Fortified with renewed strength and encouraged by a "health-inspiring atmosphere," he embarked on a planned round-trip to California, a tour he hoped would encompass not more than eighteen months. This period, for one reason or another, stretched into five years, and Beadle managed during that time to visit each of the western states and territories. Upon his return in 1873, he produced from carefully kept data a monumental and popular work, *The Undeveloped West: or, Five Years in the Territories,* a book subsequently reissued in 1877 under a new title.[10] Like Gregg, Beadle informed his reader at the outset that his was a health-seeking jaunt, and after returning to his native Hoosierdom, he concluded that he was "vastly improved in health by [his] five years of Western travel."

Although he spent much of his time in Salt Lake City, he actually preferred Denver to all other cities visited. About its attractions he said little but implied much: "Have not Greeley, Richardson, Bowles," he wrote, "and a score of lesser lights, exhausted the resources of the dictionary, in trying to tell the simple truth about its present greatness and certain future?" Their descriptions, he felt, were matchless, and he merely added, "Those are my sentiments." Such a biased affirmation by the most widely publicized invalid of the early postwar period could hardly fail to enhance Colorado's appeal or to raise greater aspirations among diseased Valley residents.

By 1876, Colorado was being flatteringly referred to as "The World's Sanitarium." Frank Fossett asserted that the state's climatic advantages and scenic attractions "are unrivaled, and have given her a world-wide reputation," and he added that "no climate on earth possesses such invigorating health renewing prop-

[10] The new title was *Western Wilds and the Men Who Redeem Them.*

erties."[11] Such assertions made observers more conscious of the mounting numbers of eastern residents who were taking advantage of the Colorado climate. A New Yorker, A. C. Wheeler, wrote in 1876:

> . . . there were long-lost and given-up victims of gout and rheumatism and phthisis, continually coming back from this dim and uncertain paradise, and suddenly appearing on Broadway, forthwith enraging everybody by their effusive health.[12]

Thoroughly impressed by what he heard and saw, Wheeler resolved to locate the fabled fount of perfect health. "Any place," he conjectured, "where life was not in continual conflict with one's environment, must be worth discovering for the benefit of the pulmonic race." Boarding a train, he traveled to the state, rambled through its many scenic parks, and finally proclaimed Manitou Springs to be the most favorable resort area in Colorado. "A pretty wide experience of watering places," he concluded, "enables me to speak with conviction, when I say that I believe this spot will in time become a national resort."

The state by 1880 definitely was living up to its advance billing. Frank Fossett in 1879 estimated that among the great number of travelers who came to the state every year "there were thousands of invalids . . . who [came] on a pilgrimage in search of health" and who were, in general, finding it. Isabella Bird also confirmed that "consumptives, asthmatics, dyspeptics, and sufferers of nervous diseases, are here in hundreds and thousands, either trying the camp cure for three or four months, or settling here permanently." And Winslow Ayer recorded in 1880, "Invalids from all parts of the world visit Colorado, and very many

[11] Frank Fossett, *Colorado: A Historical, Descriptive, and Statistical Work*, 143.

[12] A. C. Wheeler, "On the Iron Trail," *Scribner's Magazine*, Vol. XII (August, 1876), 530–39.

of them make it their permanent residence. . . . To consumptives, both in fact and tendency, Colorado has become a Mecca, without equal on the continent for salutary climatic influences."[13]

The job of advertising Colorado had been done well; its name had indeed become "great as a sanitarium," but it was the health-seeker who actually gave this designation its true meaning and significance. A. A. Hayes, Jr., himself an avid promoter of the region, admitted in 1880 that the name "sanitarium"

> has been made . . . by the sick themselves, coming of their own instinct, as it were, over the great plains, many falling by the way, but many more, after much privation, finding health and strength, and staying to build up a new State with their own labors.[14]

Resident coughers came with the early settlers and prospectors. The first recorded invalid settler, at least for the Denver area and perhaps for the entire state, was Andrew Sagendorf who arrived by ox team on November 6, 1858. He had been so ill with consumption that "boards were carried in the bottom of the wagon to build a coffin for him as it was generally believed by the others in the caravan that he would die before reaching the new country."[15] He not only recovered but spent the remaining fifty-four years of an eighty-six-year life span in helping to build up Denver. He was the first secretary of the "Aurorian Town Company" and later was instrumental in consolidating Auroria and Denver.

Others presently followed. In May, 1859, Horace Austin Tabor brought his sickly wife, Augusta, to the Cripple Creek area. While she was recovering, Tabor plunged into mining and grew exceed-

[13] Frank Fossett, *Colorado: Its Gold and Silver Mines . . . and Health and Pleasure Resorts*, 104; Isabella L. Bird, *A Lady's Life in the Rocky Mountains*, 47; J. Winslow Ayer, *Life in the Wilds of America*, 231.

[14] A. A. Hayes, Jr., *New Colorado and the Santa Fe Trail*, 184.

[15] Nolie Mumey, *History of the Early Settlements of Denver*, 77–78.

ingly wealthy; one sixty-four-dollar investment alone brought him a return of half a million dollars. He later became a prominent political figure in Colorado. Another invalid, Judge Levi H. Shepard, entered the territory in the spring of 1863. Rejected for service in the Union Army because of physical disabilities, he dissolved his law partnership, left his home in Sandusky, Ohio, and joined the movement to the Rocky Mountain gold fields. He recovered, prospered, and became a highly respected member of the bench in Colorado.[16]

The trickle of resident health-seekers before 1865 became a raging torrent after general westward emigration was resumed. The later arrivals were, in most cases, easy to distinguish from older settlers of the region; "Newcomers in Colorado"—an account attributed to Bayard Taylor—"may be recognized by the spots of blood upon their handkerchiefs."[17] So discernable and numerous were the sufferers from tuberculosis that many observers were moved to attempt crude estimates of the total number in the territory. The most generous, but obviously quite exaggerated, appraisal was made by Isabella Bird in 1879; "In travelling extensively through the Territory . . . I found that nine out of every ten settlers were cured invalids." Other estimates ranged downward from one-half to one-third, the latter constituting the general consensus. "It is a remarkable fact," a railroad advertisement stated in 1881, "that a large proportion, probably nearly one-half, of all the people now residing in Colorado were influenced in coming here, either directly or indirectly, by considerations of health." A more reliable authority, Dr. Samuel Edwin Solly, wrote in 1880: "It is often estimated that a third of the population of Colorado came for their health or that of their families, and probably the estimate is not excessive." John T. Tice,

16 Amanda M. Ellis, *Bonanza Towns: Leadville and Cripple Creek,* 3; Emma Shepard Hill, *A Dangerous Crossing and What Happened on the Other Side, vii.*

17 Titus Munson Coan, M.D., "Climate for Invalids," *Harper's New Monthly Magazine,* Vol. LVIII (March, 1879), 587.

in 1872, and Edward P. Tenney, in 1880, suggested the same figure.[18]

By 1890 there were in Denver alone thirty thousand invalids, more than one-fifth of the city's total population, who made up what was shockingly called "the one-lung army." No shame was attached to the nick-name, for as a rule, most of them were men of wealth, cultivation, and taste who took pride in their contributions to a thriving city. "There have been," Julian Ralph quoted one of them as saying in 1893:

> more important factors in the making of this unique city than most persons, even in Denver imagine. The stock and oil and gold and silver millionaires point to their operations as the cause of Denver's importance; and they are right. But importance is one thing, and good taste, good society, and progressiveness are quite different things. It was not mining that begot the taste which crowds our residence quarter with elegant dwellings, or that created a demand for clubs like the Denver Club. It was not oil that gave us college-bred men to form a Varsity Club of 120 members, or that insisted upon the decoration of the town with such hotels as ours. The influence of the invalids is seen in all this. They are New Yorkers, Bostonians, Philadelphians, New Orleans men, Englishmen—the architects, doctors, lawyers, and every sort of professional men being among them.[19]

With such numbers of them present in the city, the extent of their contributions was not surprising.

Denver was not alone in attracting an influx of health-seekers and in feeling the weight of their influence. Colorado Springs, which grew up in the 1870's, owed its origin principally to the presence of medicinal springs in a nearby glen known as Mani-

[18] Bird, *A Lady's Life*, 47–48n.; Denver and Rio Grande Railway, *Health, Wealth and Pleasure in Colorado and New Mexico*, 123; Hayes, *New Colorado*, 184; John T. Tice, *Over the Plains and on the Mountains*, 153; Tenney, *Colorado: New Homes in the West*, 40.

[19] Julian Ralph, *Our Great West: A Study of the Present Conditions*, 319. Frederick W. Pitkin, an early governor of the state, was a member of the "army." Hubert Howe Bancroft, *History of Nevada, Colorado, and Wyoming 1540–1888, Works*, XXV, 448n.

tou, an area shrouded with a score of Indian legends. Made known to Americans by Frémont, Ruxton, and other explorers, the springs were, by 1880, visited annually by "thousands of invalids," many of whom "established their dwellings about them."[20]

Two of Colorado's most renowned invalids resided in Colorado Springs, foremost of whom was James John Hagerman. When he arrived in 1881, Hagerman's financial condition was decidedly better than his health; at forty-six he was both a millionaire and a consumptive. Born in Canada, he matriculated at the University of Michigan, graduated in 1861, and went into business shortly thereafter. He acquired, between 1867 and 1879, thousands of acres of timber lands and long-term leases on rich iron-ore deposits in Michigan. Declining health accompanied his increasing fortune, and he was advised by physicians to travel for his health. After a two-year tour of European resorts, he returned to the United States and chose Colorado Springs as his new home.

Hagerman's business acumen led him into several new and profitable ventures, all of which were of great benefit to Colorado. He became the largest stockholder in the world-famous Molly Gibson mine near Aspen, and when the major railroads refused to build a trunk line into that area, he bought into the Colorado Midland Railroad Company, built the Aspen extension, and inspired the construction of service lines into other mining areas.[21] The touch of Midas deserted Hagerman in later years, however, and he eventually lost his millions in an ill-advised venture into some Pecos River projects near Carlsbad, New Mexico. He then moved to Roswell, but salvaged little from the disastrous investment. Another devastating misfortune was the humiliating removal of his son as governor of the territory by

[20] Ayer, *Life in the Wilds of America,* 233.

[21] William A. Keleher, *The Fabulous Frontier: Twelve New Mexico Items,* 169; Harvey L. Carter (ed.), *The Pikes Peak Region: A Sesquicentennial History,* 20.

Theodore Roosevelt on grounds "shot through with political intrigue." He died in Milan, Italy, in 1909, during a "travel for rest."

Helen Hunt Jackson, "the most brilliant, impetuous, and thoroughly individual woman of her time," was another of Colorado Springs's famed invalid residents. Mrs. Jackson came to the resort after a series of tragedies; an accident claimed her first husband (Edward B. Hunt) in 1863, diphtheria the last of her children in 1865, and a series of illnesses all but kindled her own funeral pyre in 1872. Believing that "climate is fate," she left her Rhode Island home, traveled first to California and then to Colorado, and finally established permanent residence at Colorado Springs in 1875. She was married to William Sharpless Jackson, a merchant of that city, in October, 1875.

Left alone after the death of her first family, Mrs. Jackson cultivated a latent literary aptitude and became an accomplished poetess and novelist before bronchial troubles set her to traveling. For her, climate alone was not fate; during her western sojourn she observed the gross mistreatment of the American Indians and was moved to the zeal of a crusading reformer. "I believe," she wrote to a friend in January, 1880, "the time is drawing near for a great change in our policy toward the Indian." Her two books, *Century of Dishonor* (1881) and *Ramona* (1884), had as their sole object the delineation of the wrongs done the aborigines, and the influence of the books was nationwide. The first brought her an appointment from the United States government as a commissioner to examine and report on "the condition and needs of the Mission Indians of California," an assignment she assumed enthusiastically and fulfilled admirably.

Misfortune struck again in 1884; a broken leg brought on a long confinement; she then contracted malaria following a change of residence to California; and a short while later a "concealed cancerous affection" which baffled her physicians made her remaining days burdensome. She passed away peacefully on

August 12, 1885, and following temporary interment in San Francisco, her body was returned to a burial place she had previously specified—"a spot near the summit of the Cheyenne Mountains, about four miles from Colorado Springs."[22]

Not all of Colorado's invalids were Hagermans and Hunts nor all its health centers a Denver or a Colorado Springs. For each person of prominence who came, there were thousands of faceless, nameless individuals. Travelers frequently mentioned seeing them but bothered little with identification. Taylor noted a "rheumatic eremite" on the opposite shore of a river he was following; Bowles spotted a "Chicago invalid" near Dalton and some twenty or thirty more scattered about in the neighborhood of Manitou; Eliza Greatorex listed a "Bavarian" from Illinois near Dayton, a "hermit invalid" at Manitou, the sweet but diseased "wife of Will" in a camp near Denver, and a "poor sick wife and mother" who had come to Colorado too late to be cured; Bickham, some invalids living in tents in Estes Park; and Hayes, "a woman who had come from the Pacific coast to camp out for her health."[23] Perhaps the most heart-rending account of an unidentified health-seeker was provided by Lady Duffus Hardy. Riding on a Pullman car en route to Colorado, she saw

> a tall, delicate-looking young man, so thin and fragile it seems as though a gust of wind would blow him out of this world into the next. He rarely speaks, but sits leaning his head upon his hand, coughing the terrible, hacking cough which tells a sad story. He is travelling in search of health . . . the more eagerly he pursues, the faster it seems to fly from him. In our mind's eye we see the phantom Death chasing him from land to land.[24]

[22] "Mrs. Helen Jackson ('H. H.')," *Century Magazine*, Vol. XXXI (December, 1885), 252, 255–56; "Helen Jackson," *The Nation*, Vol. LXI (August 20, 1885), 150.

[23] B. Taylor, *Colorado*, 94; Bowles, *Switzerland of America*, 72, 130; Greatorex, *Summer Etchings in Colorado*, 22–23, 40, 87; William D. Bickham, *From Ohio to the Rocky Mountains*, 159; Hayes, "Vacation Aspects of Colorado," *Harper's New Monthly Magazine*, Vol. LX (March, 1880), 546.

[24] Lady Duffus Hardy, *Through Cities and Prairie Lands*, 92.

Many of Colorado's myriad mineral and hot springs also became collecting points for men with diseased frames, but they were, for the most part, lesser stars in a heaven having two brilliant suns. Heywood Springs, Idaho Springs, Glenwood Springs, Pagosa Springs, and a number of others began a slow rise toward the popularity they later achieved, but none was destined to dim the luster of Denver and Colorado Springs. The post–1880 invalid population which dispersed itself among these resorts did so after Colorado had ceased, in a technical sense, to be a frontier territory. A large percentage of the invalids were proselytes, encouraged to come by railroads, doctors, or state boards of health which took over the role of advertising the state's climatic and natural attractions from early traveling laymen. When this occurred, the search for health in Colorado became highly professionalized and increasingly expensive, a trend which was to prove characteristic of the southwestern health frontier.

No portion of the health frontier passed more quickly from a semifrontier to the heavily promoted stage than southern California.[25] Already celebrated for its wonderful climate, its reputation in the early postwar years was still considerably greater than its population; but the completion of the Pacific railway in 1869 and, a few years later, the Santa Fe, made the region easily accessible and brought in annually a volume of settlers the size of which had not been seen since the gold rush.

Although a proximity to the larger segments of population and the convenience afforded by the early extension of rail service gave Colorado a temporary advantage, most health-seekers by the late 1870's showed a definite preference for the sunny Pacific coast. This came as no accident, for southern California received the most elaborate and successful promotion of any part of the salubrious Southwest. Billed as the "Italy of America," the area

[25] Southern California's health frontier has been thoroughly researched. All undocumented statements on California that follow, except as otherwise noted, are taken from John E. Baur, *The Health Seekers of Southern California.*

with the "only perfect climate in the world," the region quickly became well known throughout the eastern states for its year-round equable climate. By 1873 such towns as San Diego, Santa Barbara, and San Bernardino in the lower part of the state and Stockton and Visalia in the San Joaquin Valley were receiving wide attention as "the points most favorable for consumptives and persons subject to throat difficulties."[26] After 1880, Los Angeles, until then a struggling town with only a few score of invalids, began its its mercurial growth and in time became the "Capital of the Sanitarium Belt," the queen city of southern California invalidism.

Only briefly did the region reflect a frontier atmosphere. Health-seeking immigrants who arrived in the seventies found few conveniences or accommodations and were obliged to live in tents or wagons. But a building boom both in residences and sanatoria, one which perennially lagged behind demand, gradually alleviated housing and hospital shortages, and an intense rivalry between ambitious town builders and real estate agencies drove most communities to a saturation point by the nineties.

Like Colorado, California attracted its share of prominent invalids. Such men as Robert Louis Stevenson, Joseph Pulitzer, Andrew McNally of Rand, McNally and Company, and Philip Danforth Armour, "the world's greatest butcher," were among those who sought cures for various ailments. It was, however, the "hundreds" and "thousands" of vaguely identified valetudinarians who helped to triple the state's population between 1870 and 1900. According to one conservative estimate, at least one-fourth of this increase came as health-seekers, and "in almost every important respect—agricultural, commercial, residential, cultural—this health rush permanently changed southern California."

Colorado and California were but two of the three big resort

[26] Charles Nordhoff, *California: For Health, Pleasure, and Residence,* 110.

areas of the immediate postwar years. Texas, despite its relative inaccessibility, enjoyed a popularity among migrant invalids almost equal to that of the other two regions. First of the southwestern states to be settled by health-seekers, Texas throughout forty years of uninterrupted immigration and settlement had attracted a continuous flow of men whose hope in coming was the restoration of health. There was, in addition, a steady growth from 1821–61 of Texas' reputation for healthfulness that circulated persistently throughout America and Europe.

Response to these circulating accounts can be measured by the fruit they bore. Doran Maillard, for example, arrived from England on January 30, 1840, and acknowledged:

> In the month of November, 1839, being in delicate health, and led away by the exaggerated accounts then, as well as now, promulgated respecting Texas and the Texans, I embarked for that land of promise.[27]

Viktor Bracht, a German observer in the state during the late forties, visited thousands of his countrymen who had settled in the central Texas hill country, and wrote:

> Here the expectations of many, who came to find a healthful climate, were either surpassed or at least justified. The experiences of many German physicians have confirmed the truth of earlier reports about the climate. In truth, the healthfulness and pleasantness of the climate of this entire region far surpasses that of the northern, western, and even southern parts of the United States.[28]

To Texas in 1852 came Milton Faver, a New York City tubercular whom doctors had advised "to go West to die." Faver's insurance companies, fully expecting to have to pay a rather large indemnity, made a liberal, pre-death settlement with him and felt fortunate at having been able to escape the full amount.

[27] N. Doran Maillard, *The History of the Republic of Texas,* 2.
[28] Viktor Bracht, *Texas in 1848,* 13.

He took his benefice, "acquired ranching lands in the Big Bend country . . . married a Mexican woman, raised some half-breed children and a lot more cattle," and left an indelible mark upon "the land that renewed his life." And as a distinguished regional historian has concluded about Faver, "he did not die until age took him."[29]

From neighboring Louisiana, a former transient invalid returned to Texas in 1857 and established permanent residence. George Wilkins Kendall, consumptive editor of the New Orleans *Picayune*, bought what proved to be his final home when he purchased a ranch in the Texas county which presently bears his name. Though he commuted occasionally to his New Orleans office, he devoted much of his time to sheep raising and eventually became known as the father of that industry in Texas. He died in 1867 at Post Oak Springs, his ranch home.[30]

One of the earliest and most unique forms of promoting the physical attributes of a state also originated in Texas when in 1858 the first annual volume of the *Texas Almanac* was issued by the Galveston *News*. That one of its primary purposes was to attract settlers in general and health-seekers in particular is clearly in evidence throughout the county-by-county surveys which began in the 1858 volume. Descriptions, contributed usually by local residents in each case, employed two general criteria in assessing the resources of the counties—fertility of soils and conditions relating to health.[31]

Most writers were prone to exaggerate, or—even more typical of Texans—to brag about the salubrity of their locale. Even the transplanted Kendall depicted the mountainous regions of Comal and Blanco counties as a country

> where even the lightest bilious attacks are almost unknown, and

[29] J. Evetts Haley, *Jeff Milton: A Good Man with a Gun*, 75.
[30] W. P. Webb, *Handbook of Texas*, I, 945.
[31] *Texas Almanac for 1858*, 55–87.

where physicians are compelled to resort to other callings than their regular profession to gain a livelihood.

John H. Brown in describing Bell County wrote boastingly:

> For health, Bell is unsurpassed in this or any other State; and upon the whole, has the highest claims to the favorable considerations of newcomers. We challenge our sister counties to show twelve larger men than Bell can boast, one of whom goes to three hundred and thirty pounds.

Most favorable in appealing directly to sanitarians were county reports such as this:

> Lampasas county was settled at the Lampasas Sulphur Springs, by Mr. Moses Hughes, in 1853. Having learned of these springs, he came, seeking relief for his lady, her disease being dropsy. She soon become [sic] hearty, and from the time that it became known, hundreds flocked to this place, seeking relief from their infirmities. . . . Three years only have passed since the waters were first known, and now all the hotels are full, and hundreds are encamped out, making quite a town of camps.[32]

Thus the legend continued to grow. Before the Civil War caused a temporary stoppage, Texas' invalid traffic, though never voluminous, moved like a precision-built machine; with the restoration of peace, the mechanism needed only to be primed slightly in order to restore its prewar efficiency.

The *Almanac* responded anew in the postwar years, blazing away with generous appraisals of the state's climate. One of its writers boasted in 1868 of having known "hundreds of people from the Northern, Middle and Western States," who had immigrated into the western hill country, not one of whom had been subjected to a "seasoning" course of chills and fever. And he further remarked:

> Great numbers of invalids, especially of consumptive invalids,

[32] *Texas Almanac for 1859*, 127, 168, 177–78.

> from the other Southern States, resort to the region around San Antonio for the improvement of their health.[33]

The *Almanac* also took dead aim at the disbelieving and unconvinced. To refute a persistent rumor among people abroad that Texas was unhealthy, that the climate was excessively hot, and that foreigners ran a great risk in coming to a state so far south, an article in 1873 tersely replied:

> Nothing can be more remote from the truth, as thousands of foreigners from all parts of Europe can testify. . . . Indeed, there is no State of greater healthfulness than Texas, while many portions of the State, as Austin and San Antonio and the hilly regions farther north and west, are the resort of consumptives who almost invariably recover and live many years. It is a fact not to be gainsaid or denied, that for pulmonary complaints there is no climate in the world more favorable than that of the section we have indicated.[34]

Help came as usual from traveling laymen. William A. Bell, who spent several months in Texas on a railroad survey during 1867–68, found the glorious climate in western regions so healthy that he regarded it as far more valuable as a remedial agent than available medicines. J. H. Beadle, the well-known roving invalid, found many parts of the state to be healthy and noted that it was "a rare thing to hear any one cough." Stephen Powers, another pedestrian traveler in the 1870's, reflected: "Let a man travel six weeks in western Texas; and if he is not cured . . . of whatever ailment he has, it will be because there is no blood left in him." F. V. Hayden declared central Texas to be a paradise with excellent soil and "a climate which brings visitors for profit, pleasure, and health from all parts of the world." Walter Stevens during his tour of the Davis Mountain country in the 1880's noted that "there are springs all about which possess a whole apothecary ship of medical qualities." And on the high, dry atmosphere

[33] *Texas Almanac for 1868*, 168.

[34] *Texas Almanac* [*for 1873*] *and Emigrant's Guide to Texas*, 117–18.

of the region he commented, "It tones up weak lungs and enables the asthmatic to whoop and enjoy life."[35]

Less biased or more realistic reports indicated some apprehension about the climate of certain parts of Texas. Even the *Almanac*, though it must have been painful to the editors, occasionally felt "it ought to be acknowledged" that ague and autumnal bilious remittents frequently were to be encountered in some areas, particularly in northern Texas. Thomas North in 1870 warned newcomers to the lower Brazos, an area which had been particularly poisonous to him, to exercise the utmost care in selecting a homesite and further cautioned: "Three days residence there would suffice to bring on chills and fevers." And the implication in Power's lighthearted "Catechism for Texas Pups" is quite clear:

> [Question]: Why are many dogs in Texas naked?
> [Answer]: Because they have the ague so often they shake off all their hair.[36]

As if to balance these unsavory accounts, a number of highly exaggerated, self-perpetuating health legends circulated freely, the most persistent of which satirically suggested that it was virtually impossible to die in the Lone Star State. Some emigrants—one version of the myth began—were entering Texas via the Red River and met a very old man whose features were "seared and shrunken by the hand of time." He was rushing with all speed to the boundary of the state, and when asked the reason for such haste, he neither stopped nor paused but murmured in passing:

> "I am tired of life and of the monotony of the ages, I am weary of the slow steps of time and the dragging march of the centuries,

[35] William A. Bell, *New Tracks in North America*, I, *xvi*; Beadle, *The Undeveloped West*, 789; Stephen Powers, "Solid Days in Texas," *Overland Monthly*, Vol. VI (June, 1871), 555; F. V. Hayden, *The Great West*, 278; Walter B. Stevens, *Through Texas: A Series of Interesting Letters*, 30.

[36] *Texas Almanac for 1868*, 148; Thomas North, *Five Years in Texas*, 199; Powers, *Afoot and Alone: A Walk from Sea to Sea*, 120.

and I am hurrying out of Texas that I may find some place where people can die."[37]

More rational observers were quick to note, however, that although Texans did not enjoy perfect health, they did have a climate equal to that of any region. "Of course," J. R. Sprague wrote for the *DeBow's Review,* "there are occasional fevers in some sections, and people do die as elsewhere; but as a whole no part of the world compares with Texas for health." Or as C. H. Kent wrote in 1878: "We do not claim . . . that the fabled 'fountain of youth' pours its life-renewing waters evermore amid our hills and valleys, but we do claim that on our soil, and in our climate, a hardy and healthful population abounds."[38]

Railroads helped to enlarge the Texas health frontier and to increase its traffic. A few years after the Houston and Texas Central Railway entered Dallas, the city was reported to be a favorite collecting point for tuberculars. When the "Sunset" finally reached San Antonio in 1877, a "great army of health seekers" arrived annually in that city thereafter. And F. H. Taylor remarked in 1879:

> I never sat in a south or west bound train in Texas that I did not note some consumptive who journeyed toward the dry plains with hope and good prospect of regaining his lost heritage of health. The ranches are full of brown and bearded men, in full possession of glorious strength, who came hither under such conditions.[39]

37 Alexander E. Sweet and J. Amory Knox, *On a Mexican Mustang, Through Texas, From the Gulf to the Río Grande,* 184; for other versions of this tale see North, *Five Years in Texas,* 200, and the *Texas Almanac for 1868,* 168.

38 J. R. Sprague, "Progress and Resources of Texas," *DeBow's Review,* Vol. XXVI (April, 1859), 474; C. H. Kent, *Texas: The Future Home of the Emigrant,* 47.

39 O. W. Williams, "From Dallas to the Site of Lubbock in 1877," West Texas Historical Association *Year Book,* Vol. XV (1939), 2; Donald E. Everett, "San Antonio Welcomes the 'Sunset'—1877," *Southwestern Historical Quarterly,* Vol. LXV (July, 1961), 57; F. H. Taylor, "Through Texas," *Harper's New Monthly Magazine,* Vol. LIX (October, 1879), 714.

For the Texas-bound invalid, most roads led to central Texas. Within an approximate one-hundred-mile radius of San Antonio, at least a dozen towns or mineral springs rose to prominence between 1870 and 1880 and became celebrated as health resorts. Boerne, made popular in part by the graphic pen of George Wilkins Kendall; Austin, by the humorous "Texas Siftings" of Amory Knox; Fredericksburg, by a simple testimonial of Sidney Lanier; and Uvalde, by the residence of John Nance Garner, were among the towns which were "much frequented by invalids."[40] In addition, such water places as Lampasas Sulphur Springs, Luling Springs, and Sutherland Springs, all within easy access of the Alamo city either by rail or stage line, became important seasonal attractions, especially for large numbers who sought relief from internal afflictions.[41]

None of these locations, however, muted the cougher's call to Old Bexar, an acknowledged "Sanatarium of the West." A large floating population was a yearly expectation, and a colony of resident consumptives a recognized "institution." Of the hundreds of invalids who settled permanently in San Antonio, none was more prominent or made greater contribution to the city's commercial and cultural life than Max Krueger, German-born president of the San Antonio Machine and Supply Company.[42]

[40] Significantly, all of the men named had bronchial diseases and had sought relief in the Central Texas climate. H. F. McDanield and N. A. Taylor, *The Coming Empire; or, Two Thousand Miles in Texas on Horseback,* 144; Sweet and Knox, *Sketches from "Texas Siftings,"* 188; Sidney Lanier, *Retrospects and Prospects,* 82n.; Bascom N. Timmons, *Garner of Texas: A Personal History,* 13; and Seth Shepard McKay, "John Nance Garner," West Texas Historical Association *Year Book,* Vol. XXXVII (October, 1961), 4. Kerrville also was listed as "a considerable resort for consumptives." Mrs. Mary Jaques Marchant, *Texan Ranch Life,* 49–50. Rudolf Eickemeyer, himself a consumptive, reported in 1894 that the plaza in El Paso was "daily filled with people" who came there to mend weak lungs. Rudloph Eickemeyer, *Letters from the South-West,* 8.

[41] James L. Rock and W. I. Smith, *Southern and Western Texas Guide,* 179–83.

[42] Marchant, *Texas Ranch Life,* 44; Thomas Hughes (ed.), *G. T. T.: Gone to Texas,* 79. *Herbert Durand* (ed.), *San Antonio, Texas: The City of Missions,* 66; Lanier, *Retrospects and Prospects,* 78; Max Krueger, *Pioneer Life in Texas,*

The initials of this regionally famous corporation—SAMSCO—were, and still are, a familiar mark of identification on thousands of windmills and other machine equipment throughout the Southwest.

Improved transportation made possible the rapid emergence of a number of late nineteenth-century resorts such as Mineral Wells, Wooten Wells, and Marlin, and it also encouraged a continual flow of transient invalids to these and other more isolated areas.[43] Elliot Roosevelt, brother of President Theodore Roosevelt, in 1876–77 twice sought a climatic cure for chronic asthma at Fort McKavett; Albert B. Fall, en route in 1880 to health in New Mexico, paused for a season on a west Texas ranch in an effort to rebuild weak lungs; William Sydney Porter, who later made a fetish of anonymity as an author, began his career in Austin, whence he had come in 1885 to redeem his health; Jay Gould, unscrupulous railroad tycoon, rode his private Pullman car to El Paso in 1892 for the same reason; and C. W. Post, for whom a city on the south plains of Texas is named, attempted to recover from a nervous disorder near Fort Worth in 1885 before he returned northward and gained fame as one of America's greatest breakfast cereal manufacturers.[44]

Texas also had its share of oft-mentioned, but poorly identified, health-seekers; representative of these is this gripping account of one designated only as "Poor Tom," a sunny-tempered, golden-haired former Confederate soldier:

An Autobiography, 17; Clarence R. Wharton (ed.), *Texas Under Many Flags,* III, 81–83.

[43] One of the most isolated hot springs resorts developed during the eighties in the Big Bend country; J. O. Langford, a consumptive, was its proprietor. J. O. Langford and Fred Gipson, *Big Bend: A Homesteader's Story.*

[44] Martin L. Crimmins, "Elliot Roosevelt's Visit to Texas in 1876–77," *Southwestern Historical Quarterly,* Vol. XLVIII (October, 1944), 189; Keleher, *The Fabulous Frontier,* 182–83; Stevens, *Through Texas,* 63; *C. W. Post: A Memorial,* 8; W. P. Webb (ed.), *Handbook of Texas,* II, 396–97.

> Poor Tom! He was much wasted by the fell destroyer [consumption]; yet he was the very soul of the camp, always full of fun and jollity, and in all mud, in all miseries, kept our mess very gay. Ah! Tom, you rebel, if anywhere in this wide world, or in Texas, you still live and joke and laugh, I shake your spiritual hand across this table; but if, alas! you sleep somewhere beneath the sod, I will say, dear Tom, that no truer, manlier, or more joyous spirit ever fought in that sad, sad war, in either army.[45]

Of the large numbers of immigrants who came into Texas in the post–Civil War years, it is impossible to determine just how many were health-seekers, this despite fragmentary references to them in almost every type of literature. But, from what sources are available, it seems fairly certain that Texas ranked behind California, and possibly even Colorado, in the percentage of invalids among the total population. Much of this evidence is circumstantial but is reasonably conclusive nonetheless; for instance, in comparing descriptive adjectives used by travelers, those most used in estimating the numbers of invalids observed in Texas were "hundreds" and "large numbers" instead of the "thousands" and even "thousands upon thousands" applied in the cases of California and Colorado. Furthermore, it is certain that a large percentage of Texas' seasonal traffic was intrastate in character; temporarily disabled settlers from all parts of the state made persistent use of the resorts and watering places whenever the occasion demanded. And coastal residents, fearing summer pestilences or epidemics, frequently fled to the hill country until the threat subsided. Once restored or the danger of infection removed, these migrant invalids returned to their former homes and remained until the next wave of symptoms or warnings appeared.

Additionally, one searches almost in vain for an over-all estimate to parallel California's "one-in-four" and Colorado's "one-

[45] Powers, *Afoot and Alone,* 159

in-three" ratio between invalid and normal settlers. The absence of such an estimate becomes understandable when it is remembered that health-seeking was not the novelty in Texas that it was in other parts of the health frontier. A prolonged association with valetudinarians created only an attitude of indifference toward them in the older settled areas; even in San Antonio, most popular resort city in the state, citizens were almost "ambivalent toward these people," and some boardinghouse owners "would not permit the invalids in their establishments," fearing their diseases were communicable. And Jay Gould reveled in seldom-found privacy in El Paso, "the one place where he could . . . walk about like a plain every-day American citizen." No great building boom in either housing or sanitaria greeted the influx of eastern coughers until the late 1890's; indeed, one of Texas' oldest and most frequented mineral springs, the oil-rich Sour Lake near Houston, had only a modest commercial development before the discovery of Spindletop at the turn of the century sharply reduced its appeal as a health resort.[46] Indifference did not turn into resistance until after 1900, and the flow of immigrant invalids continued despite their casual acceptance.

This indifference did not greet sanitarians in New Mexico and Arizona; these territories struggled diligently for settlers throughout the nineteenth century and welcomed cheerfully any prospective resident regardless of motive, be it for "health, wealth, or a ruined reputation." At a time when some parts of the Southwest were being overrun with immigrants, the southern half of the old Mexican Cession, with the exception of a few old towns, was the habitat of maurading Indian bands, of crusty old prospectors, and of lawless renegades and desperadoes—a place unsafe even for sturdy pioneer famers, not to mention for enfeebled health-seekers. As such, these lands of enchantment and sunshine

[46] Everett, "San Antonio Welcomes the 'Sunset'—1877," *Southwestern Historical Quarterly*, Vol. LXV (July, 1961), 57; Stevens, *Through Texas*, 63; Jesse A. Ziegler, *Wave of the Gulf*, 147–52.

became major resort areas much later than Colorado, California, and Texas.

Travelers in the sixties and seventies, though readily cognizant of the long-acknowledged salubrity of the lower Southwest, were just as quick to recognize the real deterrents to its exploitation. Indians were the most dangerous barrier encountered. "As soon as [New Mexico] can be made safe . . . against wandering tribes of Indians," George Pine wrote in 1870, "few places offer more inducements for the emigrant." In the same year Josephine Clifford, an army wife, commented, "Could but that fearful scourge, the Apache, be removed, there are portions of [Arizona] that would soon vie . . . with the most populous sections in California." And even as late as 1878, Edward Greene, a touring botanist, noted that the Apaches in New Mexico were again "on the rampage . . . and [were] keeping all travelers and the few scattered settlers in a state of perpetual fear."[47]

Equally paralyzing was the absence of adequate transportation. Most travelers felt as Charles Clever wrote, "The climate is so unsurpassed that . . . the country needs only a railroad to develop its capabilities."[48] Finding suitable locations for rail lines, however, was no easy task, but preliminary activity had begun in this regard. General William J. Palmer, agent for the Kansas Pacific Railway spent several months in the Southwest, including a winter in Arizona, surveying possible railroad sites. His report in 1867 brought great hope and much encouragement both to his company and to prospective immigrants:

> The route throughout is singularly favored in the matter of climate. . . . For healthfulness, it is conceded to have no superior. In our engineering parties, numbering, with attaches, some 150

[47] Pine, *Beyond the West*, 126; Josephine Clifford, "Camp-Life in Arizona," *Overland Monthly*, Vol. IV (March, 1870), 247; Edward Lee Greene, "Rambles of a Botanist in New Mexico," *American Naturalist*, Vol. XII (March, 1878), 174.

[48] Charles P. Clever, *New Mexico: Her Resources; Her Necessities for Railroad Communication*, 17.

young men, and exposed to numerous hardships, there was not, either going or returning, a single case of real sickness, and all came home much heartier and more robust than when they started.[49]

For one reason or another, railroad constructions in New Mexico and Arizona lagged noticeably behind other southwestern states, and travelers continued for some time to lament their absence. Hiram C. Hodge, a traveler in Arizona during 1874–76, predicted that "when the country is opened up, and traversed by railroads, Yuma and . . . other points will of necessity become the centers of sanitariums of world-wide celebrity." And of New Mexico, L. P. Brockett conjectured in 1881, "I have no doubt that when the means of access to this country are more easy, and it is in consequence better known, it will rival or supersede [even] . . . the much vaunted paradise of Mentone as a sanitarium."[50]

Although its early resort development was slow, New Mexico enjoyed the advantage of having been explored and settled for almost three centuries; few of its physical attributes were unknown. Once the Indian and transportation barriers were broken, a flood of health-seekers poured into the territory; and the older towns, long-known mineral springs, and even newer, undeveloped sites felt the sudden impact of their numbers. "If divorce has 'made' Reno financially," Katherine Gerould once reflected,

> tuberculosis has "made" both Albuquerque and Santa Fe . . . in the same sense. . . . the endless rows of little shacks that consist chiefly of a screened porch with a bed on it, are depressing. The object of the shack is pathetically clear; and the inhabitants—hopeful or hopeless—take no trouble to beautify their surroundings.[51]

[49] William J. Palmer, *Report of the Surveys Across the Continent in 1867–68,* 109.

[50] Hiram C. Hodge, *Arizona as It Is,* 28–29; L. P. Brockett, *Our Western Empire,* 1060. Mentone was a celebrated French resort on the Mediterranean Coast.

[51] Katharine Fullerton Gerould, *The Aristocratic West,* 116.

If tuberculosis "made" those cities, a full range of afflictions "made" Las Vegas the unrivaled king of New Mexican health and pleasure resorts. Within a twenty-mile radius of the city there were mineral and hot springs too numerous to mention individually, but the one that received the greatest commercial development was Las Vegas Hot Springs, just six miles by rail from the town. Its fabulous Montezuma Hotel, the adjoining bath houses, and four-a-day train service from Las Vegas made it a favorite halfway station for passengers bound for the West Coast as well as a popular watering place for scores of invalids.[52]

Typical of the emerging centers was Eddy (now Carlsbad). Walter Stevens visited that thriving Pecos Valley community in 1892 and wrote:

> The streets of Eddy are full of people who have come to the Pecos to prolong life. This is a climate so dry that to die means to dry up, not to decay. . . . In and about Eddy are a former railroad builder from Chicago, a retired army officer, two doctors from Ft. Wayne, Ind., a retired merchant from La Cross, Wisc., another doctor from Van Wert, O., an Oakland (Ill.) merchant, a nephew of the late William H. Seward, Lincoln's Secretary of State, an Englishman and a Scotchman of means, a New Yorker, a civil engineer from St. Louis, and a real estate man from the same place.[53]

But in order to set the record straight, Stevens concluded, "It isn't true that everybody in the Pecos Valley has come for health. Occasionally there is a man who has found this a place to make money." Unfortunately, James John Hagerman, the Pecos-ruined Colorado cougher, was not one of the latter.

Mineral springs were found in every section of the state, and few, if any, escaped attention. "Since the railroad has entered New Mexico," wrote William Ritch in 1885, "from every point of the compass with lines running conveniently near to several of these springs, they are placed within easy and comfortable reach

[52] *Las Vegas Hot Springs*, 6ff.; *San Miguel County, New Mexico*, 53.
[53] Stevens, *Through Texas*, 37.

of the world. Good hotels and bath houses . . . have recently been provided for the rapidly growing demands of invalids and tourists." And in 1888, the wife of the territorial governor reported that invalids came in every train on the Pacific road with the hope of finding a new lease on life at one of the western oases.[54]

Most of New Mexico's early invalids came as unknown individuals and remained—like the "Fat Jack" described by J. H. Beadle—only vaguely but sometimes interestingly identified:

> We are off for another day's ride, with the celebrated "Fat Jack" for driver. Ten years before "Fat Jack" lived on Dayton Street, Cincinnati, and might have traveled as the "Original Living Skeleton." Some unnameable and wasting disease had reduced him to less than ninety pounds weight. He started West, began to improve, reached New Mexico, and went to driving stage, and now weighs two hundred! He is five feet four inches high, and four feet two inches around the waist.[55]

Frontier communities seldom allowed men of talent to remain undistinguished for long, and a number of former invalids quickly filled a portion of the vacuum of economic and professional leadership. At Socorro in the 1880's Russian-born, Chicago-reared John Greenwald became an eminent miller; and Illinois-born, pharmaceutically trained W. G. Hammel became a prominent brewer. At Las Vegas after 1886, Dr. Frederick E. Onley, a wheezing Ohio dentist, established a successful practice and was later elected mayor of the city; and George H. Hunker, a hacking Virginia lawyer, hung his shingle alongside that of Charles Hedgecock and thereafter helped to establish the People's Bank and Trust Company. And for the territory as a whole, at least one governor, William T. Thornton (1893–97), came from the ranks of restored invalids.[56]

[54] Ritch, *New Mexico, Historical and Industrial,* 72; Susan E. Wallace, *The Land of the Pueblos,* 9–10.

[55] Beadle, *The Undeveloped West,* 445.

[56] F. Stanley, *Socorro: The Oasis,* 205–206; F. Stanley, *The Las Vegas Story* (New Mexico), 322, 325; Frank D. Reeve, *History of New Mexico,* II, 282.

One health-seeker who entered New Mexico in the late nineteenth century eventually rose to national prominence and well-deserved infamy; that person was Albert Bacon Fall, who came to the territory in 1881 in an effort to cheat death and lived to swindle the nation.[57] Born in Kentucky, Fall shunned an inclination toward the ministry and read law under Judge William Lindsley before poor health forced him westward. After settling in Kingston, Fall became a successful lawyer, acquired more than modest ranch lands, won a United States Senate post, and in 1921 was appointed secretary of the interior by Warren G. Harding. Within two years of the appointment, Fall's double-dealings in the nation's oil reserves brought ineradicable shame to him, his party, his nation, and his state.

As in other southwestern states and territories, a number of legends circulated concerning New Mexico's climate and its effect on longevity. Perhaps the oldest and most revered tale was the one recorded by George Pine in 1870, a legend repeated earlier by the health-seeking Josiah Gregg:

> The old people of [New] Mexican towns look older than in any other country. There is a local proverb that this region is so healthy that the oldest inhabitants never die; but lean, attenuated and wrinkled, like Egyptian mummies, dry up ultimately and are blown away.[58]

Arizona also had its myths and folklore, much of which centered in the state's chief climatic attribute—sunshine. Although equable and salubrious, the climate was often hot and uncomfortable; pioneers good-naturedly referred to the area as "Nature's Turkish bath."[59] Standard among Arizonans was an oft-repeated story which depicted the territory as being literally hotter than

[57] Keleher, *The Fabulous Frontier,* 182–83.

[58] Pine, *Beyond the West,* 128; Gregg, *Commerce of the Prairies* (ed. by Moorhead) 4.

[59] Enoch Conklin, *Picturesque Arizona,* 42.

hell, a story which "everyone who ever met an Arizona man had to listen to on pain of summary punishment." The most subtle version of the tale was written by John R. Browne in 1864:

> It is said that a wicked soldier died here, and was consigned to the fiery regions below for his manifold sins; but unable to stand the rigors of the climate, sent back for his blankets.

Other legends contended:

> Everything dries; wagons dry; men dry; there is no juice left in any thing, living or dead by the close of summer. Officers and soldiers are supposed to walk about creaking; mules it is said, can only bray at midnight; and I have heard it hinted that the carcasses of cattle rattle inside their hides, and that snakes find a difficulty in bending their bodies, and horned frogs die of apoplexy. Chickens hatched at this season, as old Fort Yumers say, come out of the shell ready cooked; bacon is eaten with a spoon; and butter must stand for an hour in the sun before the flies become dry enough for use.[60]

Hot though the climate was, it achieved at an early date the reputation "of being a panacea for all ills which were aggravated by dampness; asthma, respiratory ills of all sorts, arthritis, rheumatism and so on."[61] Physicians at the isolated military posts reported that climatic diseases were almost unknown, conspicuous among the missing being malaria and chronic diarrhea. Dr. John Stark, post surgeon at Fort Mojave in 1866, stated:

> The atmosphere, of course, is very dry, dew never being seen. . . . I hazard nothing in saying that a more healthful and healing climate for those laboring under that great destroyer, phthisis, could be desired. These cases seldom present themselves, and

[60] Charles E. Sajous (ed.), *Annual of the Universal Sciences,* D–19; J. Ross Browne, "A Tour Through Arizona," *Harper's New Monthly Magazine,* Vol. XXIX (October, 1864), 571; J. Ross Browne, *Adventures in the Apache Country,* 56–57.

[61] Edward H. Peplow, Jr., *History of Arizona,* II, 355.

> then only among emigrants. . . . I am now stationed here about two years and have not had a death among the troops during that period; evidence that good health is our epidemic.[62]

One of the earliest, and certainly the most legendary, tuberculars to take advantage of that arid climate was John H. "Doc" Holliday.[63] Fast becoming a prominent Atlanta dentist in 1872, Holliday was forced to leave Georgia because of failing health, and by the time he reached Texas in 1873, he had begun to leave a trail of "wanted" posters behind him. Never one to let law and order stand in the way of self interest, he managed to stay only one jump ahead of peace officers as he moved from Texas to Oklahoma, back to Texas, to Kansas, and finally to Arizona.

Although there definitely was something wrong with his lungs, there apparently was nothing wrong with his stomach; along with a number of killings he is credited with consuming an average of two or three quarts of the most expensive whisky every day. He managed to survive on this meager fare for fourteen years—an excellent testimonial indeed for the restorative qualities of Arizona's climate (or the life-giving potency of good liquor).

Holliday's case history closed in 1887 at a health resort in Glenwood Springs, Colorado, in what was a desperate, but unsuccessful, attempt to halt the rapid decline in his health. Following his death, a friend of long standing, Wyatt Earp, summed up Holliday's career with this fitting epitaph:

> Doc was a dentist whom necessity had made a gambler; a gentleman whom disease had made a frontier vagabond; a philosopher whom life had made a caustic wit; a long, lean, ash-blond

[62] Quoted in B. Silliman, "On Some of the Mining Districts of Arizona near the Río Colorado, with Remarks on the Climate, etc.," *The Journal of American Science and Arts,* [n.s.] Vol. XLI (May, 1866), 291.

[63] John Myers Myers, *Doc Holliday,* 256; see also Pat Jahns, *The Frontier World of Doc Holliday.*

> fellow nearly dead with consumption, and at the same time the most skillful gambler and the nerviest, speediest, deadliest man with a six-gun I ever saw.[64]

All other Sunshine State invalids seem insignificant by comparison despite Holliday's negligible contributions to the state. But more significant, if less notorious, contributions were made by such coughers as A. P. K. Safford, who served as territorial governor of Arizona (1869–77); Hiram C. Hodge, a prerailroad traveler who became one of the state's most effective promoters; Thomas Carson, a world traveler and sportsman who became a prominent southwestern rancher; and Charles DeGroff, owner of the first hotel in Tucson designed to cater to the growing community of health-seekers who "forced themselves" upon the city after 1880.[65]

Tucson, because of enterprising men like DeGroff, became one of Arizona's major collecting points for health- and pleasure-seekers. By 1897, Arcadia, a small nearby village, contained "a coterie of wealthy, cultured Easterners" whose robust appearances made it difficult "to imagine they were ever in delicate health." And other eastern business men frequently sent their "sickly sons" to Tucson or to nearby towns and ranches, hoping (and succeeding in the vast majority of cases) to transform them into "strong, vigorous, self-respecting young men."[66]

Had the number of people immigrating into Arizona and New

64 Myers, *Doc Holliday,* 256. Myers quoted from the San Francisco *Weekly Examiner,* August, 1896.

65 Richard J. Hinton, *The Hand-Book to Arizona,* 323; Frank C. Lockwood, *Arizona Characters,* 112; H. C. Hodge, *Arizona as It Is, v;* Thomas Carson, *Ranching, Sport and Travel,* 42ff.; and J. George Hilzinger, *Treasure Land: A Story,* 57. Hilzinger also was a tubercular in search of a climate cure.

66 Hilzinger, *Treasure Land,* 56. Phoenix also was a focal point for tuberculars. Robert W. Craig, M.D., "Climatography of Arizona, with Especial Reference to the Climatic Treatment of Pulmonary Tuberculosis," *Journal of the American Medical Association,* Vol. XXXVIII (January 25, 1902), 229; Peplow, *History of Arizona,* II, 370.

Mexico been greater, these territories easily could have ranked at the very top of nineteenth-century resort areas. Invalidism accounted for a large percentage of their populations, tourism for a substantial portion of their revenues.[67] More important, the multitude of watering places, winter resorts, retirement centers, and guest ranches which presently dot both regions strongly suggests that the climatic appeal of the lower southwest has been more sustaining than those of even the most popular of the earlier resort states.

Population numbers have never been a problem to Utah and Nevada, the two remaining states on the Southwest health frontier. The search for health has had only a marginal effect on the growth of their populations. People going to the Mormon State have done so largely to find a saint's haven, not a cougher's paradise, and those to the Silver State essentially to find diversion, not to regain health. Still, both states offer a variety of climatic and physical attractions, and each can point to a small number of health-seekers. F. V. Hayden, who visited both areas in the seventies, regarded the climate of Utah as being "favorable to consumption and bronchial troubles," and J. H. Beadle, who spent two seasons in Salt Lake City, stated that the climate relieved his respiratory distresses. Hayden's approval of Nevada's "remarkably healthy and invigorating" climate was later supplemented by Mark Twain's observations near Lake Tahoe:

> I know a man who went there to die. But he made a failure of it. He was a skeleton when he came, and could barely stand. . . . Three months later he was sleeping out of doors regularly, eating all he could hold . . . and chasing game over mountains three thousand feet high for recreation. And he was a skeleton no

[67] A resident physician estimated that half of the people in New Mexico had come there for health reasons. H. B. Masten, M.D., "New Mexico as a Health Resort," *New York Medical Journal*, Vol. LXXVII (September 6, 1902), 415.

longer, but weighed part of a ton. This is no fancy sketch, but the truth. His disease was consumption. I confidently commend his experience to other skeletons.[68]

Gradually the frontier disappeared, and with it, much of the uncultured, undeveloped characteristics of an untamed environment. Such a turning point for the western health frontier came between 1880 and 1890; invalid traffic during that period ceased to be sporadic and spontaneous and became persistent and promoted. The growth of commercialized resorts was a chief characteristic of the new era and a sophisticated, scientific study of climatology a major rationalization. Scrupulous promoters succeeded in turning the search for health into big business at a time when physicians could prescribe nothing more dependable than a change of climate as a cure for even the simplest diseases.

Not to be overlooked as an enduring characteristic was the none too subtle fact that the nation had a serious health problem. The overcrowded slums of eastern industrial cities joined the Mississippi Valley as a major contributor to the army of "walking death" which trekked westward at every opportunity and in every type of conveyance. The gravest blight was tuberculosis, a "white plague" that besieged young and old, rich and poor, sophisticated and uncultured with undiscriminating disaster. Climate alone seemed to be effective against this disease, and for those gripped by the lethal bug, nothing was as reassuring as, or more beneficial than, a change of residence to one of the southwestern states—to nature's sanatorium.

[68] Hayden, *The Great West,* 304, 320; Beadle, *The Undeveloped West,* 329; Mark Twain, *Roughing It,* 171.

VI. *Consumption and Climatology*

CONSUMPTION, according to Samuel Hopkins Adams, was "the real race suicide" of the nineteenth century:

> It causes more deaths, more suffering and sorrow, and a greater economic loss, than any agency within the whole range of human afflictions. This nation, thanks to its vast open spaces, suffers less than many others, yet of the 75,000,000 living Americans, 8,000,000 at least must inevitably die from this cause; some authorities put the estimate as high as 10,000,000.

Although Adams was more of a muckraker than a medical observer, his conclusions were confirmed by nearly every physician of his era. Even as early as 1875, Dr. Joseph W. Howe used almost the same terms and figures in analyzing the tuberculosis problem, calling the disease the "scourge of the human race" and estimating that one-tenth of the "civilized people in the temperate regions" would be carried off by its ravages. Dr. Samuel A. Fisk, equally concerned, noted in 1886 that 91,500 Americans died every year from pulmonary consumption, a disease which accounted for "12 out of every 100 deaths in the United States." And Dr. Samuel S. Wallian, in 1900, estimated that "the standing army of tubercle stricken invalids" approximated 1,200,000 and that in all probability an equal number of undetected, incipient cases also existed. Thus the white plague was, indeed, as Dr. A. L. Benedict wrote, "the chief lieutenant of Death."[1]

Tuberculosis had been a problem in every previous century, but a horrifying increase in the number of afflictions from the malady developed in the second half of the nineteenth century. The causes were not hard to identify. Both Howe and Adams, though a quarter-century apart in their observations, declared that conditions incident to rapid urbanization and industrialization were the chief contributors. Crowded, poorly ventilated, and unsanitary tenement or slum houses were ready breeding grounds for phthisis; overworked, undernourished, and debilitated factory workers and miners were easy prey for the silent working parasitic germ. Yet a full chorus of criticism and an endless legion of social workers in the late nineteenth century did little to alleviate these distressingly infectious conditions; by 1900, death ratios from tuberculosis were largely unchanged, and physicians were grimly predicting that "100 years of hard united work" lay ahead before phthisis could be brought under control.[2]

If the industrial revolution had its manifold sins, it also possessed a few compensatory virtues. Since the only agent powerful enough to stay the executioner's hand—Nature—was found in its most salubrious trappings in the remote Southwest, railroads provided easier access to the region and an improved standard of living a broader financial base for individual travel. Moreover, the expansion of communication media made possible the widest dis-

[1] Samuel Hopkins Adams, "Tuberculosis: The Real Race Suicide," *McClure's Magazine,* Vol. XXIV (January, 1905), 234; Joseph W. Howe, M.D., *Winter Homes for Invalids,* 5–6; Samuel A. Fisk, M.D., "Colorado as a Winter Sanitarium," *Popular Science Monthly,* Vol. XXVIII (March, 1886), 668; Samuel Spencer Wallian, M.D., "The Search for Health," *Junior Munsey,* Vol. VIII (1900), 463; A. L. Benedict, M.D., "Consumption Considered as a Contagious Disease," *Popular Science Monthly,* Vol. XLVIII (November, 1895), 39.

[2] B. S. Moore, M.D., "The Experience of Syracuse, N.Y., with the Compulsory Tuberculin Tests," *Journal of the American Medical Association,* Vol. XXXVIII (January 25, 1902), 229.

semination of information not only on southwestern climates but on the latest scientific and medical discoveries as well.

A promising break-through in the treatment of tuberculosis occurred in 1882 when a German scientist, Robert Koch, discovered and isolated the tubercule bacillus. Clinicians, however, grappled fruitlessly thereafter in an attempt to find an agent which would end the germ's parasitic existence in the human body; in fact, Koch's discovery, though of undoubted importance to the eventual control of tuberculosis, was regarded by many practitioners as having retarded rather than furthered the treatment of the disease. Too much emphasis was placed on the germ itself, too little on the people afflicted by it.[3] Numbers of new "specifics" were produced, each specific claiming to be the cure to end all cures, but each fell quickly into disrepute. Accordingly, "the world's experts," meeting at an international tuberculosis convention in 1900, without a dissenting voice formally announced that "*there is no known medicinal specific* for this fatal and increasing malady, and . . . the only hope of cure, in its curable stages, is the climatic cure."[4]

Throughout the nineteenth century, the failure of formal medicine served increasingly to strengthen the faith of health-seekers in the physical rewards of a suitable climate, and although they continually sought relief in the sunny Southwest for a variety of afflictions, tuberculosis accounted for at least 80 per cent of all invalid immigration. Most emigrants were dispatched by physicians who, admittedly, were overwhelmed by the disease and saw no solution other than travel-cure therapeutics. Tireless, dedicated, but constantly frustrated in their efforts to check the spread of phthisis, many doctors worked until they too became

[3] Walter R. Bett and others, *The History and Conquest of Common Diseases*, 109; Arnold C. Klebs, M.D., "The Home Treatment of Pulmonary Tuberculosis," *Transactions of the American Climatological Association*, Vol. XVII (1901), 207.

[4] Wallian, "The Search for Health," *Junior Munsey*, Vol. VIII (1900) 463.

tubercular and were forced to join that ever expanding corps of wanderers who searched for health.

The utilization of climate therapeutics by a rather large group of consumptive physicians was a significant trend in the early postwar years, one which added a professional touch to the development of the health frontier. Driven from their practices and studies in widely separated parts of the East, these men dispersed throughout the Southwest and became staunch defenders of the regions in which they found renewed health. From their experiences as convalescents and their investigations as climatotherapists they were able to compile an elaborate documentary on the climatic attributes of the Southwest and to offer encouragement to the "hundreds of thousands of citizens of this great Republic" who annually sought "healing in a change of climate."[5]

The movement of diseased doctors to the frontier began around 1870. Among the first of them was Dr. Isaac Davis, an English-born, decorated veteran of the Crimean War. He emigrated to New Jersey in 1859 and lived there until the outbreak of the Civil War. Severely wounded at Bull Run, Davis suffered thereafter from nervous prostration, an affliction which was subsequently agitated by an intense application to his medical studies. After graduating from New York University Medical College, he practiced briefly in Brooklyn until poor health forced him westward. He arrived at Manitou Springs, Colorado, on February 19, 1871, built the first house ever occupied as a dwelling at that soon to be famous resort, recovered his health, and treated countless invalids; he later became a prominent druggist and real estate promoter.[6]

Two of Colorado's most prominent nineteenth-century doctors joined Davis in that state within the next three years. In 1874, a fellow countryman, London-born-and-educated Dr. Samuel Ed-

[5] B. James, *American Resorts,* 17.

[6] Henry Dudley Teetor, "A Pioneer of Manitou Springs," *Magazine of Western History,* Vol. XIII (December, 1890), 159–61.

win Solly, established permanent residence at nearby Colorado Springs.[7] Destined to become one of the most important western climatologists, Solly began his study of the climatic treatment of pulmonary diseases at the age of eighteen when a breakdown in his own health occasioned a tour of Egypt, the Riviera, and Switzerland. Following a successful practice of a few years in London, a second and more severe breakdown brought him to Colorado at the age of thirty. Plunging immediately into a study of Rocky Mountain climate, Solly became in time an acknowledged authority on climatology and was the author of many books, pamphlets, and articles which brought him widespread recognition from medical fraternities and societies. None of these organizations gave him more honors or brought him greater respect for his labors than the American Climatological Association, a society for which he served as president in 1895.

A colleague of Solly's in the Association, and one of that organization's original numbers, was Dr. Charles Denison.[8] An 1869 graduate of the University of Vermont and an 1873 victim of pulmonary hemorrhages at Hartford, Connecticut, Denison moved westward in an effort to arrest his affliction, paused briefly in San Antonio, Texas, and settled finally at Denver, Colorado, the "Queen City of the Plains." Fully recovered after a short residence, he engaged in a highly successful practice of medicine, taught for fourteen years as professor of diseases of the chest and climatology in the University of Denver, and served thereafter as professor emeritus until his death in 1909. Like Solly and other physicians who regained lost health in Colorado, Denison was a devout disciple of the climate of the region; and like his English associate, he was an enthusiastic contributor to and an honored president (1890) of the American Climatological Association.

[7] James A. Hart, M.D., "In Memoriam: Samuel Edwin Solly, M.D., M.R.C.S.," *Transactions of the American Climatological Association,* Vol. XXIII (1907), *xxv–xxvii.*

[8] "Charles Denison: [In Memoriam]," *Transactions of the American Climatological Association,* Vol. XXIV (1908), xxiii.

Harvard-trained Dr. Samuel A. Fisk, another prolific nineteenth-century author on western climates and a frequent contributor to the Association's annual bulletin, also recovered his health and practiced in Colorado but did not locate there permanently. A tubercular at twenty-four, Fisk became, after 1881, the vagabond of western physicians, traveling extensively throughout the health frontier in "search of a suitable climate."[9] His lifelong quest took him, among other places, to Minnesota, Utah, and southern California, but Colorado, quite early in his wanderings, pleased him most. Fisk opened an office in Denver in 1883 and practiced in that city until 1898, when a new and recurring illness forced him to abandon the profession. Adrift again, he sought relief at sea-level resorts and by walking "hundreds upon hundreds of miles" in the open air. Many of his later writings were composed "while [his] feet [were] making the dust fly."

Collectively, Solly, Denison, and Fisk made a contribution to the development of western climatology equal to that of all the other physicians who worked in that field of study. Their opinions were respected, their investigations studied, and their advice sought by all who endorsed climatic therapeutics for respiratory diseases. And significantly, each of them was, in effect, living documentation for their copious testimonials on the efficacy of western climates.

The convictions of this Colorado triumvirate were shared and supplemented by a large number of health-seeking physicians who came to the Southwest between 1870 and 1900. Among the best-known of these invalid (and sometimes transient) doctors were James A. Hart, J. W. Brannon, and Jeremiah T. Eskridge of Colorado;[10] Francis W. Gallagher, S. T. Lowrie, and Eugene

[9] "A Search for a Suitable Climate," *Transactions of the American Climatological Association*, Vol. XXIII (1907), 40–52. Fisk also served as president of the association in 1902.

[10] Physicians, interestingly enough, freely admitted and openly discussed

M. Littlejohn of Texas;[11] Paul M. Carrington, Edward E. Elliott, and E. S. Bullock of New Mexico;[12] B. G. McPhail, Mark A. Rodgers, and E. Payne Palmer of Arizona;[13] and William A. Edwards and H. S. Orme of California.[14] The works of these men were much more localized in character; each chose that particular area which seemed most beneficial for his own afflictions, and each in turn became an ardent student (and promoter) of the climate of his region. The products of their studies provoked many lively discussions on the corresponding and contrasting climatic elements of the various regions of the Southwest; and as a result, a large amount of statistical information was made available on every part of the health frontier. In time, a serious effort was made to reduce these findings to a science of medical climatology.

Dr. Charles Denison was the first to conceive a formal, systematic study of climatic effects on chronic diseases. For him, necessity evoked the expedient. Aware of the "growing and very

their previous status as invalids; see for example Hart, "In Memoriam: Samuel Edwin Solly," *Transactions of the American Climatological Association*, Vol. XXIII (1907), *xxvi;* Carl Ruedi, M.D., "A Comparison of the Winter Health-Resorts in the Alps with Some Places in the Rocky Mountains of Colorado," *Transactions of the American Climatological Association*, Vol. X (1893–94), 41; "Obituary: Dr. Jeremiah T. Eskridge," *ibid.*, Vol. XVIII (1902), *xxxi.*

11 Gallagher, "The Rocky Mountain Region, Especially New Mexico," *New York Medical Record*, Vol. XLV (March 10, 1894), 300; Pat Ireland Nixon, M.D., *A Century of Medicine in San Antonio*, 154–55; Littlejohn, M. D., "San Antonio and Southwest Texas as a Winter Resort," *New York Medical Record*, Vol. XLII (November 19, 1892), 588.

12 Carrington, "Economic Housing of Consumptives, with Special Reference to the Southwest," *New York Medical Record*, Vol. LXI (April 10, 1909), 423; Elliott, "A Practical View of Tent Life in the Southwest," *New York Medical Journal*, Vol. LXXXIV (October 6, 1906), 685; E. Bullock, M.D., "The Southwest as a Resort for Pulmonary Patients," *Journal of the Outdoor Life*, Vol. III (1906–1907), 47.

13 McPhail, "Special Report on Climatic Influence and Health Resorts of the Western Territories," *Transactions of the Medical Society of Virginia*, Vol. II (1879), 395; Rodgers, "The Climate of Arizona," *Transactions of the American Climatological Association*, Vol. XII (1896), 105; E. Palmer, "Phoenix, Arizona, as a Health Resort for Tuberculosis Patients," *New York Medical Journal*, Vol. LXXII (November 17, 1900), 852.

14 Edwards, "Littoral California," *Transactions of the American Climatological Association*, Vol. XVIII (1902), 127, 135; see also William A. Edwards and Beatrice Harraden, *Two Health-Seekers in Southern California*.

general distrust among physicians" of drugs alone in the treatment of diseases and appalled at "our failures individually to stem the tide of death," he called for a "united effort" from those who were "devoted to the prolongation of life and the adaptation of climate to the needs of invalids." All practitioners, he felt sure, were aware of the relieving qualities of a generous climate, but the evidence of such relief was intangible to the masses since it was "only scattered in the experience of invalids who have found health in strange lands, or in the transient conclusions of physicians who have, at odd moments, and so imperfectly, investigated the subject." To aid future health-seekers, he suggested the creation

> of a Climatic Association, composed of physicians interested in such labor, and especially representatives from the health resorts of America, . . . it should be their work to gather statistics of all climates, familiarize themselves with the details of their special labors, and to tabulate all the results of the journeyings of invalids in America from now henceforth. . . . Through a central council or bureau of medical advisers, . . . advice could be given as to the choice of climate, mode of life needed, etc., etc. This association should always seek to prevent the *useless* and encourage the *useful* migrations of invalids, and continually watch over the journeyings of their patrons.[15]

Although Denison presented the idea in 1873 to a selected group of sixty friends and physicians and received generally enthusiastic responses, eleven years elapsed before such an organization was formed.

The intervening years were not idle ones; a fairly large volume of material dealing with western climates was published in various medical journals throughout the United States and Europe. From a representative sampling of these articles, it is possible to determine what early physicians regarded as most important in climatic therapeutics. In 1874, Professor Cheever of the Uni-

15 *The Best Welfare of Invalids Seeking the Benefits of Climate,* etc., 7–8.

versity of Michigan, a consumptive in search of a cure in Colorado, wrote that it was difficult to determine which of the properties of Rocky Mountain atmosphere were the most beneficial. But he observed pragmatically that he, in common with other consumptives there, was "much *better* when the air [was] ordinarily dry, and much *worse* when a damp east wind" prevailed. He noted also that "the rarity of the air" forced lungs "to expand more fully to supply the system, and hence aerations as well as circulation" were promoted. Dr. Denison, in 1876, added that the greatest benefits from Colorado's "stimulating and tonic climate" came only to those "*who* [were] *able to be out of doors . . .* as *indoor* life [had] no special advantages." And, in 1877, Dr. Hermann Weber, a well-known German physician, concurred that dry air and soil and sunshine were the most important attributes of a healthy climate, and agreed that outdoor living, for those adapted to it, was most helpful.[16]

Reports also came from other sections in the western territories. In 1877, Dr. J. J. Jones, an invalid who found Colorado lacking in "the imperative equability of temperature [and] necessary warmth," wrote that he preferred "the high and dry atmosphere" and "the equable and temperate climate" of New Mexico, conditions which permitted invalids "unending out door exercise." Then in 1879, Dr. B. G. McPhail, a tubercular writing for the Virginia Medical Society, declared that consumptives fared best in an atmosphere which was free from dust and moisture and blessed with abundant sunlight so that daily outdoor exercise was permissible. He also concluded that "a low altitude [was] . . . generally most favorable." These conditions he thought to be present in their most generous proportions in a belt lying

[16] Prof. Cheever, "Colorado as a Sanitarium," *The Peninsular Journal of Medicine*, Vol. X (February, 1874), 55–56; Denison, "Report on the Climate of Colorado and Its Relation to Pulmonary Disease," *Transactions of the American Medical Association*, Vol. XXVII (1876), 462; Weber, "Manitou in Colorado (U.S.A.): A Health Resort in Consumption," *The Lancet*, Vol. II (August 4, 1877), 156–57.

between the 32 degrees and 35 degrees latitude, extending from the "valley of the Rio Grande to the Pacific." And Mrs. Gulnare Garrison, sent to Southwest Texas by her husband, Dr. J. B. Garrison of Arkansas, proved the doctor's firm belief that tent life in the dry, pure air of Texas would benefit even "the most delicately-constituted" consumptive.[17]

In addition to these short treatises in professional magazines, a few penetrating studies appeared in print during the same period. Dr. Samuel Solly, in a perceptive summary of the climate at Manitou Springs, concluded that mountainous air was much to be preferred to sea-level air; the greater dryness, the decreases in pressure on the lungs from a rarefied air, and the almost constant sunshine of higher elevations during both winter and summer provided a "tonic influence" on the invalid which he seldom felt in lower elevations. Dr. Joseph W. Howe, somewhat more cautious than Solly, agreed that exercise in a dry, warm atmosphere was essential to successful convalescence but warned that elevated climates were not suitable for all patients. He suggested that care be taken in selecting a proper location for each particular case; some invalids, he declared, improved more rapidly in coastal surroundings.[18]

Despite Howe's admonitions, the early medical consensus ran in favor of elevated climates. Important contributions to this theory were made in 1880 by Doctors Charles Denison (Colorado) and H. P. Gatchell (Georgia), whose conclusions were based on several years of experience in treating respiratory diseases in different sections of the country.[19]

[17] Jones, "New Mexico as a Health Resort for Consumptives," *Medical and Surgical Reporter*, Vol. XXXVII (September 15, 1877), 201; McPhail, "Special Report on Climatic Influence and Health Resorts of the Western Territories," *Transactions of The Medical Society of Virginia*, Vol. II (1879), 398. Gulnare Garrison, "Southwestern Texas as a Health Resort," *Medical and Surgical Reporter*, Vol. XLIV (January 22, 1881), 91.

[18] Solly, *Manitou, Colorado, U.S.A., Its Mineral Waters and Climate*, 31–32; Howe, *Winter Homes for Invalids*, 8–9.

[19] Denison, *Rocky Mountain Health Resorts: an Analytical Study of High*

Thus the most important factor in the study of climatology was the air. If it was pure—that is, free of moisture, dust, pollen, and the like—it was thought also to be free of the infectious miasmata so prevalent in the atmosphere of the Mississippi Valley and eastern United States. Elevation and sunshine were regarded as important sterilizing agents and life in the out-of-doors as the best method of obtaining a maximum of hygenic values from atmospheric elements.

Enough interest arose by 1884 to warrant the establishment of an association whose purpose it was to study and synthesize the collective findings of interested physicians. In that year, forty-two prominent doctors met at Washington, D.C., on May 3 and formally launched the American Climatological Association, an organization destined to publish its transactions annually for more than half a century. Its constitutionally stated objective was "the study of climatology and the diseases of the respiratory organs."[20] Only two of the original members, Charles Denison and H. S. Orme were western physicians; twenty-seven listed New York as their permanent residences. A highly respected New Yorker, Dr. Alfred L. Loomis, was chosen as the society's first president—a fitting selection, since at an earlier date he personally had realized the climatic benefits for consumption in an Adirondack retreat.

Illness prevented Loomis from presiding at the first annual meeting, and a Bostonian, Vice-President Frederick I. Knight, delivered the opening address in words and thoughts which must have sounded familiar to Dr. Denison. "Our professional brethren," he began,

> will probably look to the minutes of our first meeting as to the preface of a book, to see what reason we can give for our exist-

Altitudes in Relation to the Arrest of Chronic Pulmonary Disease, 162ff.; Gatchell, *The Invalid's Guide: Where to Go in Search of Health,* 16–17.

20 "The Constitution and By-Laws of the American Climatological Association," *Transactions of the American Climatological Association,* Vol. I (1884), 89.

> ence . . . . Our answer is that we believe that more can be accomplished by a small body of thoroughly interested men, working independently in a limited field, rather than as a part of a great combination . . . we feel that the interests of climatology will be better served by its isolation. . . .
>
> One of our first objects . . . should be to place before the general profession, for every-day use, well-known and indispensable facts about climate.[21]

In the years that followed, this group of dedicated climatologists admirably fulfilled Knight's commission. Indeed, two of the six papers presented at the initial session, Charles Denison's "Dryness and Elevation the Most Important Elements in Treating Phthisis" and Frank Donaldson's "City Air and City Life Injurious to Consumptives," not only predicated the future work of the association but also demonstrated its firm grasp of the problems surrounding the treatment of the "white plague." And although the charter membership was predominantly eastern, the scope of the organization's study was nationwide. The number of western climatologists increased, however, and the volume of their climatic studies multiplied throughout the years until the association developed a recognizable western orientation.

There was an unfortunate drawback to the work of the association; its findings, although always definitive, were published only once a year. In consequence, reports on some of the regions of the Southwest were much delayed, and the void often had to be filled from other sources. Many of the professional medical journals devoted a part of each issue to climatology, but none of them attempted to specialize on the subject. By combining all printed evidence, however, physicians could put together a reasonably comprehensive and fairly useful set of facts on the climates of most portions of the health frontier.

Students of Colorado's climate were most laudatory of the

[21] "The Opening Address," *Transactions of the American Climatological Association,* Vol. I, (1884), 2.

lands lying between the frigid Continental Divide and the heated Plains in the eastern part of the state. Here the elevation ranged downward from 8,500 to 4,000 feet above sea level, and the meteorological and physical attributes of the region varied sufficiently to meet the demands of all types of invalids.[22] The atmosphere was regarded as pure, rarefied, and aseptic, containing neither the dust nor the moisture mortally feared by consumptives. Moist Pacific winds, cooled and depleted by their passage over intervening mountain ranges, deposited no more than sixteen inches of rainfall each year, the greater portion of which fell during the spring and summer months. Soils, porous and gravelly to a great depth, were constantly dry and gave "forth no noxious vapors." Thus, Colorado, except for an occasional case of rheumatism or mountain fever, was adjudged to be almost exempt from the deadly infestations of the Mississippi Basin.[23]

The most striking phenomenon of the Centennial State's climate was the unusual amount of "clear, pleasant weather [and] bright sunshine, especially during the winter months." Fewer than sixty days each year were cloudy, and the rarefied, subhumid atmosphere permitted a maximum penetration of health-giving rays from the sun even on chilled or wintry days. The greatest annoyances encountered were infrequent "great and rapid changes in temperature." Although always cool and frequently cold, the atmosphere occasionally suffered an extreme variation from a sudden blast of polar air, a fact which rendered the climate unequable and at times even unpredictable. With this exception, physicians claimed for Colorado "a remarkable combi-

[22] Walter A. Jayne, M.D., "The Climate of Colorado and Its Effects," *Transactions of the American Climatological Association*, Vol. V (1888), 55–56; Solly, "Treatment of Pulmonary Consumption by Residence in Colorado as Exemplified by the Analysis of 141 Cases," *ibid.*, Vol. VII (1890), 131–33.

[23] Charles Fox Gardiner, M.D., "Light and Air in the Treatment of Consumption in Colorado," *Transactions of the American Climatological Association*, Vol. XV (1899), 25; See also Henry B. Baker, "Relations of Certain Meteorological Conditions to Diseases of the Lungs and Air-Passages in Colorado," *ibid.*, Vol. VII (1890), 210–238.

nation of those climatic conditions most desirable for an invalid wishing to live as much as possible out-of-doors"—an abundance of sunlight and pure air, "the most powerful weapon[s] now known with which to fight and conquer" tuberculosis.[24]

The same mountainous network which played such a vital role in determining Colorado's climate also imposed its influence on parts of two adjoining states, Utah and New Mexico. Physicians in Utah were particularly pleased with the Great Salt Lake Basin, a region so isolated that it had a "climate distinctively *local* and peculiarly its own."[25] The Basin, averaging 4,300 feet in elevation, was encompassed on the north and east by the Wasatch Range and on the south and west by desert lands. Carefully kept statistics revealed that despite a slightly heavier annual rainfall, the area had an average relative humidity lower than that of Colorado, but this condition was delimited somewhat by a higher than normal content of atmospheric moisture during the winter months, the most critical time of the year for tuberculars. Westerly winds, dried before reaching the Basin by their passage over arid deserts, were thought to possess "tonic properties of sea air" after they had mingled with vapors arising from the Great Salt Lake. Endemic fevers were virtually nonexistent, and if present at all, were brought in by transients. Temperatures ranged from cool to very cold, but this factor was modified somewhat by the absence of high winds. A maximum number of days could be spent outdoors in glorious sunlight, and invigorating salt water baths in the lake were available for those who desired them.

What was true of Colorado and Utah climates was largely true

24 Solly, "Invalids Suited for Treatment at Colorado Springs," *Transactions of the American Climatological Association,* Vol. V (1888) 24; also, "An Invalid's Day in Colorado Springs," *ibid.,* Vol. IV (1887), 175; Gardiner, "Light and Air in the Treatment of Consumption in Colorado," *ibid.,* Vol. XV (1899), 19.

25 A. C. Standart, M.D., "The Climate of the Great Salt Lake Basin," *Transactions of the American Climatological Association,* Vol. VII (1890), 76; see also McPhail, "Special Report on Climatic Influence and Health Resorts of the Western Territories," *Transactions of the Medical Society of Virginia,* Vol. II (1879), 399–401.

of northern New Mexico; it too had a Rocky Mountain environment. Certain advantages, however, were claimed for the land of enchantment by some of its climatological students. Since it was farther south, its temperatures were more moderate and its winters relatively free from the "piercing cruel wind" which sometimes plagued northern areas.[26] For the discerning invalid, altitudes varying from three thousand to ten thousand feet were available; it was almost possible to have summer in winter and winter in summer if locations were judiciously and appropriately selected.

Nature made New Mexico the crossroads between two distinctly different climatic zones. The climate of southern New Mexico, far more consistent with that of western Texas and Arizona than of Colorado and Utah, belonged to a region known as the "Arid Southwest," a land which was excessively dry and perpetually baked by sunshine. Summers, though hot, were regarded as pleasant, winters as being "without the sting of the colder North which drives the invalid from out-of-door life to the confinement of ill-ventilated rooms." As proof of its healthfulness, physicians pointed repeatedly to the absence of phthisis among the native population despite its indigent appearance and total disregard of sanitary habits.[27]

Only one feature detracted from the "general excellence" of New Mexico's climate; high winds in the late winter and early spring months brought annoying sand or dust storms, the wind and dust both being more severe in areas unprotected by high mountains. "Such storms," one doctor wrote, "have an undoubted effect on the nervous system of patients, most of whom become irritable and cross on the second day and almost unbearable on

[26] Gallagher, "The Rocky Mountain Region, Especially New Mexico," *New York Medical Record,* Vol. XLV (March 10, 1894), 301.

[27] Gallagher, "The Climate of New Mexico," *ibid.,* Vol. XLIX (June 13, 1896), 848; James H. Worth, M.D., "The Climate of New Mexico as Viewed by the Medical Fraternity There," *Transactions of the American Climatological Association,* Vol. VII (1890–91), 286.

the third. When the storm subsides the fact is clearly recorded on the smiling and cheerful faces of everyone."[28]

For patients who preferred year-round summer climates at lower elevations, Southwest Texas also offered pleasing prospects. Nearly all of the lands west of Austin and San Antonio, including the Edwards Plateau and the trans-Pecos Plains plus the southern portions of the *Llano Estacado* and the Texas Rocky Mountains, were regarded as proverbially salubrious and particularly adapted to respiratory diseases. According to serious-minded (and biased) students of the region's climate, it was for "three-fourths of the year . . . unsurpassed by any country in all that contributes to the health, comfort, or pleasure of its inhabitants." The sandstorms which plagued New Mexico and the Texas Panhandle were far less frequent, because of the direction of prevailing winds and the natural protection afforded by a few mountain ranges. Summers were "delightful" and only because of their length were "considered objectionable in any sense"; temperatures, admittedly hot during the day, were so reduced at night as to require light bed coverings. Winters rarely were colder than 20 degrees Fahrenheit, and were made uncomfortable only by the sporadic appearance of one of the state's famed "northers," the chilly but dry "tail-end of a Dakota blizzard."[29] Even this phenomenon did not appear unheralded, but gave ample notice of its coming, and only a slight, advance alteration in wearing apparel was needed to turn its numbing winds into a "stimulating, highly electrical, and healthful" experience. And as for

28 Carrington, "The Climate of New Mexico—Nature's Sanatorium for Consumptives," *Transactions of the American Climatological Association*, Vol. XXIII (1907), 76.

29 M. K. Taylor, "The Climate of Southwestern Texas and Its Advantages as a Winter Health Resort," *Transactions of the American Climatological Association*, Vol. V (1888), 213–14; E. W. Schauffler, M.D., "The Climate of El Paso, Texas," *ibid.*, Vol. III (1886), 210; R. W. Knox, M.D., "Texas Climate in the Trans-Pecos Region," *New York Medical Record*, Vol. LV (April 1, 1899), 463; Milton J. Bleim, M.D., "The Place of Southwest Texas in Climate Therapeutics," *Medical Century*, Vol. II (December, 1903), 525.

humidity, a most important consideration for consumptives, Southwest Texas compared favorably with all but Arizona, in the lower, more arid climatic zone.

Arizona, a land of "frightful chasms, dark and gloomy canyons, massive mountains, rolling plains, rich and fertile valleys, arid wastes, and beautiful mountain vales," was a panorama of nature both in her wildest topographical temper and her most extreme meteorological mood. So varied was the Arizona terrain that Dr. Mark A. Rodgers described it in 1896 as a "washboard," possessing a contour so peculiar that plains were interspersed between six mountain chains. The summits of these mountains constituted the general level of the wind currents, and moisture usually condensed at the higher elevations and rarely fell in the intervening valleys. Thus, the hilly regions were covered with great forests; the lower mesas were arid wastes.[30]

Northern Arizona, much more elevated than the southern portion of the state, possessed a typically mountainous environment. Cool and inviting in the summer months, it became cold and forbidding during the winter. During the five or six "desirable" months, residents of the area enjoyed a dry, equable, and cloudless atmosphere—the air charged with the soothing aroma of pine forests. Chilling wintry winds, however, brought snows and discomfitures and forced the more timorous invalids to descend the mountains to a warmer climate.[31]

Arizona physicians claimed for southern Arizona "the finest winter climate of any section of the North American Continent." One rabid proponent commented rather convincingly in November, 1893:

> Here can be found an unsurpassed number of sunshiny days and dryness of atmosphere—the days comfortably warm, the nights

30 "The Climate of Arizona," *Transactions of the American Climatological Association*, Vol. XII (1896), 88, 93.

31 William G. Burns, M.D., "Climate of Arizona," *ibid.*, Vol. XVIII (1902), 242.

> cool and permitting refreshing sleep. No dews, no fogs, no rapid changes from heat to cold, no decaying vegetation, no rivers, pools, or lakes germinating poisonous miasms—evenness of temperature and pure water.[32]

Winters may have been pleasant, but summers were not. During the three or four hottest months, it was not uncommon at midday and early afternoon for the thermometer to hover between 105 and 110 degrees Fahrenheit, with only slight relief anticipated after sundown.[33] Yet, because of an almost total lack of moisture in the atmosphere a temperature of 110 degrees was not regarded as unbearable. In fact, sunstrokes were rare and fevers virtually unknown, and the hot sun literally baked the tubercule bacillus from the consumptive's body.

Southern California—all the essential climatic elements being considered—did not belong in the same health frontier with such states as Colorado, Utah, Texas, New Mexico, and Arizona; and it was, as a matter of practice, frequently listed as a separate climatic zone. An elongated "climatological peninsula," it stretches southward from Santa Barbara to San Diego, bordered on the west by the Pacific Ocean and protected from the arid deserts on the east by the foothills of the Sierra Nevada Mountains. One of the controlling factors in California's climate is the cold Alaskan current, which moves northward just off southern California sending its cooling sea breezes over an almost parched coastline.[34] Because of its proximity to the ocean, southern California possesses fewer of the more healthful attributes normally associated with the Rocky Mountain and arid-Southwest regions.

[32] William W. Hibbard, M.D., "The Climate of Arizona," *New York Medical Record,* Vol. XLIII (January 28, 1893), 111.

[33] Robert W. Craig, "Climatography of Arizona, With Especial Reference to the Climatic Treatment of Pulmonary Tuberculosis," *Journal of the American Medical Association,* Vol. XXXVIII (January 25, 1902), 230.

[34] C. F. McGahan, M.D., "The Climate of the South and Southwest," *Transactions of the American Climatological Association,* Vol. XXV (1909), 99; Edwards, "Littoral California," *ibid.,* Vol. XVII (1902), 123.

Physicians agreed that the climate on the coast of California was suitable only for a minority of tubercular cases. Moisture-laden Pacific winds kept the humidity quite high during most of the year; heavy coastal fogs frequently obscured the warming rays of the sun; sporadic rains, some of which continued for a week at a time, drove invalids indoors for indefinite periods; and "occasional stiff winds" during the fall and early winter months rendered unpleasant an otherwise equable temperature.[35] But in spite of these drawbacks, coastal towns in southern California were overrun with wheezing consumptives, a majority of whom seemed always to convalesce satisfactorily.

Where the coastal areas were hot and muggy, the "foothills" to the east were temperate and moderately dry. Fogs were less troublesome, fewer days each year were marred by rain and high winds, and temperatures were far more equable, thermometers seldom registering below 32 degrees Fahrenheit. And although the mountains of southern California were not as dry and cloudless as the barren lands of Arizona, New Mexico, and Texas, professional adherents of that more western region maintained that it had "as nearly a perfect climate as can be found anywhere."[36] A multitude of health-seekers between 1870 and 1900 obviously agreed with them.

An understandable amount of particularism emerged from these studies. Dr. George Abbott described it best, in 1902, when he commented that it seemed to be "the inalienable right of a climatologist to inhale his native climate and exhale the same in a syllabic chain, more or less at variance with the thoughts and observations of his fellows in other climates, but almost always with the approbations of those who dwell near him." Such indeed

35 Orme, "Climate of Southern California," *Transactions of the American Climatological Association,* Vol. IV (1887), 142–55; Norman Bridge, M.D., "The Climate of Southern California," *ibid.,* Vol. XVII (1901), 86–88.

36 C. A. Sanborn, M.D., "The Climate of the Eastern Foothills of Southern California," *ibid.,* Vol. XVIII (1902), 95.

was the case; yet it was difficult to refute a doctor's exhortations on the healthfulness of a location, be it at sea level or mountain top, when he himself had recovered in its climate. As such, each state or territory in the Southwest developed its own group of heralds, and each at one time or another was declared in baroque and biased affirmations to be unexcelled as a health resort.[37]

This lively, good-natured discussion between neighboring localities was a continuing, harmless affair, but in comparative studies of the broader climatic zones, particularism was ardently expressed and often vehemently defended. Because there were significantly variations in the combination of climatic elements found in the different regions, there was an intelligible basis for serious debate on the subject of the most suitable climate for consumptives. All physicians were agreed on the advisability of a dry, sun-drenched atmosphere, but after two decades of serious climatological study there was no general accord on elevation as an essential factor for a successful convalescence. Elevation to the defenders of the arid Southwest meant a colder environment and a rarefied atmosphere, both of which were dangerous to advanced cases of tuberculosis and especially to hemorrhaging lungs. But to the advocates of the Rocky Mountain zone, an altitude wisely chosen meant reduced atmospheric pressure on a diseased chest, a factor which permitted freer breathing with less strain on delicate, inflamed lung tissues. Sharp, give-and-take discussions on this subject occasionally provoked a militancy seldom observed among the cultured followers of Hippocratic ethics.[38]

[37] Abbott, "Southern California Foot Hills," *ibid.*, Vol. XVIII (1902), 96. Typical of these rabid appraisals are those of B. P. Anderson, M.D., "Colorado as a Health Resort," *New York Medical Record*, Vol. XXXIII (March 17, 1888), 314–15; George Halley, M.D., "New Mexico as a Health Resort," *Kansas City Medical Record*, Vol. V (February, 1888), 41–44; and C. L. G. Anderson, M.D., "Arizona as a Health Resort," *New York Medical Record*, Vol. XXXVIII (July 5, 1890), 8–10.

[38] Solly, "The Comparative Merits of Resorts in New Mexico, Colorado, and Arizona," *Transactions of the American Climatological Association*, Vol.

Statistics, though they actually settled few arguments, ran in favor of higher elevations. By analyzing some eight thousand cases of consumption treated by climatotherapy, Dr. Solly demonstrated to his satisfaction that the number of improved cases rose in direct proportion to altitude. "The percentage of improvement," he wrote in 1897:

> among those who took sea-voyages was 54 per cent.; in lowland climates 57 per cent.; in lowland desert climates 65 per cent.; while in altitudes the improvement runs up to 77 per cent. . . . Therefore, while the desert air of Arizona will cure more cases of consumption than the sea air of the coast, say of southern California, yet it will not cure as large a proportion as will the mountain air.[39]

Basic to the debates on elevation was the recognized but confounding fact that a part of those who journeyed into the mountains received no benefit at all, and this was true for even a greater number of health travelers who sought relief at lower altitudes. Still more confusing was the fact that opposite effects often were realized in the same climate by invalids who were afflicted with identical respiratory ailments at approximately the same stage of development; some would recoved quickly and return to robust health while others would decline slowly and perish. Why this was the case, no one knew for certain. It was the most pressing problem facing climatologists in the late nineteenth century, and there were many urgent appeals made by eastern practitioners for a clearer, more definitive stand on the question of where to send which patient for the best results and why.[40]

XIII (1897), 171–185; for Solly's determined defense of elevated climates see his discussions following: W. M. Yandell, M.D., "The Preferable Attributes of Climate for Consumption, as Applied to the Winters in Southern New Mexico, Southern Arizona, and Western Texas," *ibid.*, Vol. VII (1890), 98–99; and Bridge, "The Climate of Southern California," *ibid.*, Vol. XVII (1901), 93.

39 Solly, "The Comparative Merits of Resorts in New Mexico, Colorado, and Arizona," *ibid.*, Vol. XIII (1897), 178.

40 B. James, *American Resorts,* 156; James B. Walker, M.D., "Presidential Address: Some of the Difficulties of Climato-Therapy," *ibid.*, Vol. XII (1896), 6.

Perhaps the simplest answer was provided by Dr. Austin Flint, who recommended colder climates for consumptives who suffered more during the summer and warmer climates for those who fared worse in the winter.[41] Though his advice was practical, most physicians regarded the selection of a proper climate as being far more complex than this. "It is almost impossible," wrote C. L. G. Anderson in 1890, "to designate the exact points for each patient."[42] To begin with, patients in the last stages of phthisis were encouraged to remain at home where proper attention could be shown them and where they might live out their remaining days among friends and in happy surroundings. Tuberculars whose cases were complicated by heart trouble or by acute nervous disorders were warned to avoid extremes in weather and altitude. Advanced cases of consumption were also warned against residences at higher elevations because of the increased danger of hemorrhages in rarefied atmospheres, and were advised instead to seek the warmth of the lower valleys and mesas (though not necessarily in the arid Southwest). Persons with slight or primary cases were directed to seek locations which seemed best suited for both their constitutions and their afflictions and to be prepared for a residence of indefinite length. Finally, a good part of the selection of a preferred location was left to the invalid himself, for such things as physical stamina, distance to be traveled, and expense to be incurred were important factors to be considered in each case.

Ordinarily, climatotherapy was thought of as relating almost exclusively to tuberculosis; this was logical since it was the disease of the vast majority of health-seekers. But there were other afflictions which responded to residence in a favorable climate, particularly asthma, hay fever, rheumatism, certain skin diseases,

[41] Quoted in Cheever, "Colorado as a Sanitarium," *The Peninsular Journal of Medicine,* Vol. X (February, 1874), 56.

[42] "Arizona as a Health Resort," *New York Medical Record,* Vol. XXXVIII (March 17, 1888), 10.

and some internal disorders. Asthma and hay fever sufferers frequently found grateful and almost immediate relief by removing to a subhumid climate; rheumatics benefited either by a residence in a warm, dry atmosphere or by bathing regularly in a hot or warm spring. Eczema, psoriasis, and acne, among other common skin diseases, were often favorably affected by a dry, elevated location. And infections of the kidney responded to climatic influences in regions where soils were constantly dry and the days perennially sunny.[43]

Also highly regarded in the treatment of many diseases were natural mineral waters, the analysis of which became an important adjunct to the study of climatology. Doctors were none too certain how these natural agents acted in or on the human body, but they were convinced that many medicinal waters *did* have alterative effects on certain afflictions and ought, therefore, to be thoroughly examined so that their use might be wisely prescribed.[44]

Most of the resulting analyses were too complex and the accompanying comparisons between American and European spas too vague to be of value to anyone but trained physicians, but in time, a meaningful association of certain types of water with specific diseases emerged. For example, Dr. Bushrod James, in terms that even the layman could comprehend, listed alkaline waters as being effective against respiratory, genitourinary, malarial, and diabetic afflictions; salines in cases of scrofula, syphilis, gout, malaria, and catarrhal affections; sulphur waters in liver, respiratory, and skin diseases; chalybeate (ferrous and carbonic

[43] Knox, "Texas Climate in the Trans-Pecos Region," *ibid.*, Vol. LV (April 1, 1899), 463; H. A. Lemen, M.D., "The Influence of the Climate of Colorado on Asthma," *First Annual Report* of the State Board of Health of the State of Colorado (1877), 72; L. Duncan Bulkley, M.D., "Climate as It Affects the Skin and Its Diseases," *Transactions of the American Climatological Association*, Vol. XV (1899), 115; James B. Walker, "Some Remarks on Climate and Renal Diseases," *ibid.*, Vol. XV (1899), 102.

[44] T. G. Horn, "Report on the Mineral Springs of Colorado," *First Annual Report* of the State Board of Health of the State of Colorado (1877), 52.

acid) solutions for deficiencies of the blood such as anemia and chlorosis; calcic waters (with salts of lime or gypsum) for dyspepsia, cystitis, and diabetes; sulphurates (with sodium or magnesium) for constipation and stomach disorders; and thermal waters (with or without chemical agents) for rheumatism, gout, paralysis, and certain skin eruptions.[45]

Fortunately for the growth of the southwestern health frontier, the middle and southern Rockies were abundantly blessed with such waters, and many of the larger mineral springs promptly became teeming resort centers with facilities which rivaled the better-known eastern spas. Manitou Springs, Colorado, for example, was frequently called the "Saratoga of the West," and was even favorably compared to the internationally famous Davos-Platz health resort in Switzerland.[46]

The qualified but unquestioned success of climatic therapeutics was a godsend to consumptives and a boon to the medical profession. Once doomed to early graves, a majority of those afflicted with phthisis could look forward at least to a modest prolongation of their lives, if not to a permanent cure, by a residence in the salubrious Southwest; and doctors, once members of an enigmatic and internally disordered fraternity, now found their practices punctuated by new-found respect and professional harmony. Faith in climatic treatment became so universal that most patients accepted with unreserved approval a physician's charge to seek a more favorable environment; many, dis-

[45] B. James, *American Resorts,* 129–34; see also Coan, "American Mineral Springs," *Chautauquan,* Vol. VII (June, 1887), 543–46; Albert C. Peale, M.R., "The Classification of American Mineral Waters," *Transactions of the American Climatological Association,* Vol. IV (1887),156–66; and Guy Hinsdale, M.D., "Some Analogous European and American Mineral Springs," *ibid.,* Vol. XVII (1901), 263–65.

[46] Clinton Wagner, M.D., "Colorado Springs and Davos-Platz, as Winter Health Resorts, Compared," *New York Medical Record,* Vol. XXXII (October 29, 1887), 567–70; Ruedi, "A Comparison of the Winter Health-Resorts in the Alps with Some Places in the Rocky Mountains of Colorado," *Transactions of the American Climatological Association,* Vol. X (1893–94), 28–42.

eased or not, surged westward without waiting to be told to do so. And many doctors confidently dispatched their patients (sometimes quite indiscriminately) to a region they regarded as having been providentially created "for the betterment of the human race."[47]

Despite a general acceptance of climatic therapeutics, the medical fraternity as a whole was "lamentably ignorant of the principles of climatology, and sadly careless and ignorant in their application."[48] Admonished by western physicians to let phthisics come early and remain indefinitely, eastern practitioners were often cruelly lax in following this rule, and a large group of "came too late" invalids tore deeply into the once-heartening ratios of successful convalescences. Another substantial group, told by their medical advisers at home that a few months' residence would suffice in most cases, left the Southwest prematurely to become inevitably a lonely, pitiable statistic in "the silent halls of death."[49]

More appalling to doctors in the West was the fact that many of their eastern constituents refused to familiarize themselves with the available climatic studies before sending their patients to a particular location. In a rare moment of wry humor, Solly introduced one of his frequent papers before the Climatological Association by recalling a story told of a distinguished, but apparently uninformed, consultant that a patient once called to see:

> The servant who answered the door inquired if it was a matter of great importance for the patient to see the doctor, as he was much engaged. "No," said the patient, "I only wished to know whether he would recommend me to go to Aix la Chapelle." "I

47 George M. Kellogg, M.D., "New Mexico as a Health Resort," *Journal of the American Medical Association,* Vol. XXVII (September 12, 1896), 583.

48 Solly, "Presidential Address: The Principles of Medical Climatology," *Transactions of the American Climatological Association,* Vol. XI (1895), 1.

49 See the article by Sherman G. Bonney, M.D., "When Should the Consumptive Residing in Colorado be Permitted to Return Home?" *ibid.,* Vol. XVIII (1902), 203–207.

can tell you that he would not, because this is his Aix le Bains day."[50]

Dr. E. Payne Palmer, a consumptive who was himself a victim of poorly informed advisers, found that patients were sent to Arizona from all parts of the country without being properly informed as to the peculiarities of the climate. "Judging from those facts," Palmer concluded regretfully, "I take for granted that there are hundreds of our best physicians, over the country, that know little or nothing of either the place or the climate."[51] Such professional nonchalance was bound to work unnecessary hardship on those who were ill-suited to the rigors of Arizona's inferno-like atmosphere.

This anomalous situation—the acceptance of the principles but an indifference toward their technical application—was undoubtedly a product of the unknowable aspects of medical climatology. Although men like Solly, Fisk, Denison, Ruedi, and Orme made valiant efforts to render the study as precisely scientific as possible, they actually fell far short of that goal. The uncertainties which continually shrouded the work of the climatotherapist were exposed most graphically by Dr. James B. Walker of Philadelphia in 1896 before the American Climatological Association. He declared that a decade or more of intensified study had proved incontrovertibly that climate was not a fixed entity, that there still was a lack of definite information on the elements which affect health directly, and that the perplexing difficulty of selecting the correct climate for each individual case would undoubtedly remain unresolved for some time to come.[52]

The general public, then and now, may have kept its faith in

[50] Solly, "The Comparative Merits of Resorts in New Mexico, Colorado, and Arizona," *ibid.*, Vol. XIII (1897), 172.

[51] "Phoenix, Arizona, as a Health Resort for Tuberculous Patients," *New York Medical Journal*, Vol. LXXII (November 17, 1900), 852.

[52] "Presidential Address: Some of the Difficulties of Climato-Therapy," *Transactions of the American Climatological Association*, Vol. XII (1896), 3–8.

climate unshaken, but formal studies on the subject declined rapidly after 1900, particularly in the medical schools throughout the country.[53] Increasing attention was shown instead to bacteriological science, a field of study which in time was to place the doctor but one step lower than the angels in healing the major infirmities of mankind. Climatology was thereafter relegated to the realm of the psuedo-sciences, hardly a fitting denouement for so serious a discipline and its unrelenting disciples.

One permanent feature of the age of climatology, other than the unshakable faith of the public, was the establishment of a large number of resort centers in the Southwest. While physicians attempted to reduce medical climatology to an exact science, enterprising businessmen attempted to capitalize on the credulity (born of desperation) of great numbers of health-travelers. Powerful agencies aided the growth of the major resorts; "the attractive and seductive advertising matter," issued by state boards of immigration and health, by railroads, as well as by the larger health resorts, often played the determining role in helping an invalid choose one location over another. To this end, some physicians also became addicted to the financially prudent art of promoting fashionable centers of health and culture.

53 Solly, "Climatology as a Study in the Medical Schools," *ibid.*, Vol. XX (1904), 7–13.

VII. *The Great Resort Centers, 1870-1900*

THE GROWTH of the great resort centers in the Southwest was the product of many factors. Certainly the *sine qua non* was the sanitarian, for perceptive promoters sought always to cater to his needs and to appeal to his tastes. But the qualifications for a suitable resort location were dictated by certain natural conditions; a favorable climate or a reputable mineral springs was absolutely essential to the success of any health resort, and a combination of both gave more assurance of greater and prolonged acceptance. After these in importance came artificial considerations, such as adequate accommodations, medical attention, good food, recreational facilities, and amiable companionship.[1] By providing these services and conveniences and by playing on the credulity of men who were determined to find a health-restoring environment, enterprising resort developers were able to turn the search for health into a business of fabulous dimensions. Their handiwork remains even today as the most recognizable product of nineteenth-century invalidism.

Businessmen were but one of the interest groups at work in developing the resorts of the Southwest; other powerful and influential agencies also became prominently associated with ad-

[1]E. L. Godkin, "Summer Hotels," *The Nation,* Vol. XLI (September 11, 1884), 217–18; Edward O. Otis, M.D., "Some Observations on Health Resorts," *Journal of the American Medical Association,* Vol. VI (March 20, 1886), 316.

vertising the health attractions and facilities of the various states. For example, the efforts of official boards of health (like the one in Colorado) or of immigration (like that of New Mexico) cannot be minimized. The men behind these organizations recognized two pertinent aspects of a heavy invalid traffic, both of which were useful in state development. First, the money spent on health greatly supplemented a state's income; second, each invalid was potentially a permanent resident. The leading citizens in New Mexico were especially sensitive and alert to these facts, and they seldom missed an opportunity to publicize any testimonial which might attract invalids or, for that matter, to propose any business venture which might interest investors.[2]

Not to be overlooked as a major factor of growth was the influence exerted by railroads. Actually, the well-endowed, better-situated resorts emerged concomitantly with the development of rail transportation; indeed, a surprising number of the more famous western spas were part and parcel of railroad promotion and planning. For example, the fabulous Del Monte at Monterey, California, first of the great resort hotels in the West, was constructed in 1880 by the Southern Pacific; then, in 1882, the Atchison, Topeka and Santa Fe opened its lavish Montezuma Hotel at Las Vegas Hot Springs, New Mexico; and finally, the Denver and Rio Grande built the famous Antlers Hotel at Colorado Springs, Colorado, in 1883.[3] These as well as countless other lesser resorts owed a great debt to the coming of the iron horse.

It is inconsequential which resort center developed first or which became the most famous; facilities arose in direct pro-

[2] New Mexico succeeded very well for a time in enticing capital "thither for investment, and a great number of enterprises sprang up in almost every direction. The 'boom,' however, fell almost as rapidly as it arose . . . owing to a lack of resources in [that] Southwest region." Its salubrious climate thereafter remained its most appealing resource. Adolf Francis Alphonse Bandelier, "Why New Mexico Does Not Flourish, *The Nation*, Vol. XLII (January 28, 1886), 70–71.

[3] Earl Pomeroy, *In Search of the Golden West: The Tourist in Western America*, 19–23; *Las Vegas Hot Springs*, 6.

portion to demand, and each center persisted as long as there were health-seekers or excursionists to frequent it. But it is a matter of no little importance to note that the larger developments swiftly became centers of resort for classes, not masses, and many of them became veritable little social and cultural oases for the parvenu and hotel-dwelling rich.[4] The hands of the resort promoters were clearly visible in this trend, for after a time only the more remote, less frequented, or strictly marginal establishments made appeals directly to the general public.

The demand for resort accommodations was exceptionally heavy along the southern Pacific Coast and in the central Rocky Mountain regions. A great portion of the yearly invalid and vacationing traffic thronged into these areas and swelled, often to unmanageable proportions, the populations in and around the larger cities and mineral springs. And while climatologists debated the efficacy of the various climatic attributes of the two regions, town and resort builders plunged headlong into the task of attracting and providing accommodations for an ever increasing volume of valetudinarians who seemed oblivious to (or at least unconcerned with) the professional controversies.

John E. Baur, in a perceptive and scholarly study, has proved incontestably that the post–Civil War health frontier in southern California was a consciously promoted one.[5] Nearly every town of any size in the lower part of the state owed either its origin or its principal growth to the machinations and forthright planning of civic leaders who were courageous enough to gamble the future of their cities on "the promise of health alone." Although the region as a whole had its "king of the boosters" in Charles Nordhoff and its weathervane on the business potential of invalid

[4] For an interesting article on this subject see Charles Deming, "Changes in Summer Migration," *The Nation*, Vol. LIII, (September 17, 1891), 210–11.

[5] Here again, the research and ideas used in describing California are those of the author cited. See particularly the chapter entitled "Town Builders," in his *Health Seekers of Southern California*.

and excursion trade in Charles Dudley Warner,[6] nothing can detract from the resourcefulness of grass-roots promoters like D. M. Berry of Pasadena, Nathaniel C. Carter of Sierra Madre, Dr. Francis Pottenger of Monrovia, Douglas Gunn of San Diego, J. A. Johnson of Santa Barbara, and Myron H. Crofts of San Bernardino.

Perhaps the two cities most reflective of successful advertising as applied to potential health resorts were San Diego and Santa Barbara. Douglas Gunn, ubiquitous editor of the San Diego *Union*, began as early as 1868 to publicize that city's healthful climate and to point out to local merchants the dollar and cents value of resort traffic. Responding to Gunn's enthusiasm and sound business acumen, investors began a flurry of construction which produced fourteen hotels by 1871, at least two of which were considered "first class" establishments.

Advertisements aimed directly at the nation's invalid classes continued during the seventies at such a pace that San Diego's hostelries and residential areas soon were overrun with hopeful consumptives. For a decade, health-seekers made up the majority of the newcomers who crowded into the city; but thereafter improved transportation and increased commercial opportunities brought a different type of immigrant who in time cut sharply into the proportion of sickly people present in the population. The health trade nonetheless continued for an indefinite period to make a significant contribution to the "Bay 'n Climate" city's rising prosperity, and the construction of sanatoria in the nineties by Drs. Peter Remondino, Robert J. Gregg, and William A. Edwards relieved some of the pressure on public housing. Thus by capitalizing at an early date upon the sanatory search for health, San Diegans were able to "build" a thriving city with a diversified economy by 1890.

[6] Typical of the promotional work of Nordhoff and Warner are Nordhoff, *California: for Health, Pleasure, and Residence;* and Charles Dudley Warner, "The Outlook of Southern California," *Harper's New Monthly Magazine,* Vol. LXXXII (January, 1891), 167–89.

Another editor, J. A. Johnson of the Santa Barbara *Press*, took the lead in propagandizing the glorious climate of his city. With an energy unmatched even by the indefatigable Douglas Gunn, Johnson toured America in a sort of "crusade to inform a sickly world of hope from the Far West." The results of his efforts were equally unmatched; "a veritable human inundation [came] down upon Santa Barbara," and real estate values and business profits soared for the first time in the city's history.

Barbarenos, however, overbuilt and overspeculated. Houses soon became vacant, stores and saloons unfrequented. Not even the incomparable Arlington Hotel could retain the larger portion of the seasonal traffic which deserted Santa Barbara every year during the summer months for cities in the East or even for the more northerly San Francisco, and the city's budding health trade might have died had not Santa Barbara become a "refuge for the rich and retired." After a time, the city fathers reoriented their planning, and took pride in the coming of highly educated Yankees, people who "were of 'the better class,' refined, traveled, and usually well off financially,"—who would keep the economy stable until the coming of the next winter season.

The winter traffic might well be anticipated, but it scarcely could be accommodated even when all southern California's facilities were engaged simultaneously at the task. As late as 1905, a retired army surgeon, C. H. Alden, wrote:

> The number of winter residents and of tourists is now so great as to tax the ability of the railroads to transport them from and to the East, and hotels and boarding houses are multiplying in all the principal places. As far as can be learned, the number of consumptives coming to this region has not sensibly diminished.[7]

But by that time, the number of immigrants and sojourners of all types had increased to a point where invalids were less notice-

[7] "Some Southern California Health Resorts," *Transactions of the American Climatological Association*, Vol. XXI (1905), 44.

able. Invalidism had, however, already played its role in the development of the state and had left such monuments as the Hotel Del Monte at Monterey, the Hotel Raymond at Pasadena, the Hotel del Coronado at San Diego, the Cliff House at San Francisco, and a score of less pretentious hostelries as reminders of the once-constant search for health in those remote parts of the American Southwest. And if the excursionist or vacationer now occupied those stately rooms, it would not have been surprising if he were awakened on occasion by the faint cries of invalid predecessors long deceased or by the muted boasts of climate promoters only recently, but never completely, silenced.

Southern California's foremost competitor for the invalid's dollar was Colorado. In many respects the two regions were climatic complements; one afforded the health-seeker a haven in winter at sea level, the other a resort in summer at higher altitudes. Yet neither area was publicly tolerant of the other; in fact, both at times were quite uncompromising in making appeals to the nation's valetudinarians. Much of this competitive spirit can be explained by the economic factor involved, but a reliance on this fact alone does a gross injustice to well-intentioned climatotherapists who regarded the climate of the Rockies as vastly superior to that of all other areas. Thus, the influence of medical men was much more conspicuous in the development of a resort industry in Colorado than in California.

The most prominent of these medical promoters were none other than Colorado's renowned professional trio, Drs. Denison and Fisk of Denver and Solly of Colorado Springs. Their influence was so great that hardly anyone could speak authoritatively on the state's attractions without making a direct reference to at least one of them. Respected everywhere within the medical fraternity, quoted extensively in all types of lay promotion, and published widely in both public and professional literature, they were the logical leaders of the Centennial State's propagandizing parade.

Although these men were far from alone in advertising Colorado's resort facilities, they, more than any other promotional group, led the assault on California's claim to having the more appealing climate. Solly, in his customary role as the chief defender of elevated climates, repeatedly warned that the high moisture content of Pacific winds was dangerous to most consumptives. Fisk, the itinerant cougher who wrote from personal experience, also was critical of California's "high relative humidity" as well as its cold, nasty, and depressing fogs, its greater annual rainfall, and its occasional dust storms. And even the dignified, ever tolerant Denison once wrote that restless Colorado invalids frequently caught the "California fever" during the winter months, but that after one season's visit they were back again regretting that they had ever left the rejuvenating Rockies.[8]

Fundamental to the growth of Colorado's invalid and tourist trade, and of far greater concern to resort developers, was a combination of almost irresistible natural features. Nature had blessed the state not only with an invigorating climate but also with an array of beautiful parks and glens and a number of valuable medicinal springs. The old Jefferson Territory was an easy region to advertise; indeed, after reviewing some of the pictorial literature which circulated during that time, it is difficult to understand how anyone, who was bent on traveling, could resist the urge to see Colorado's scenic wonders.[9]

Quick to recognize the immense potential of all these natural attractions were such men as William N. Byer, editor of Colorado's first newspaper; William J. Palmer, president of the Denver and Rio Grande Railway; Dr. T. G. Horn, member of the

[8] Fisk, "Some Observations on Southern California," *ibid.*, Vol. XVII (1901), 82–83; Denison, M.D., "The Mineral Springs of Colorado," *ibid.*, Vol. VI (1889), 244.

[9] See especially William M. Thayer, *Marvels of the New West.*

Colorado State Board of Health; and Frank Fossett, chronicler-historian of the early development of the state.

William Byer arrived at Denver on April 21, 1859, in a rush, founded and published the first number of the *Rocky Mountain News* the very next day, and then spent the remainder of his professional life as an energetic promoter of his adopted city. As a civic leader, he was a champion of decency and justice (sometimes at the risk of his own safety) in that typically lawless frontier town, but as a business observer he recognized quite early the role Denver was playing as an entrepôt for invalids and tourists. One of Byer's contemporaries wrote for instance that "no less than thirty-nine thousand visitors . . . registered at Denver public houses" in a three months' period during 1878, and that often even the upper floors of vacant warehouses had to be appropriated by innkeepers to accommodate the overflow.[10]

This deluge of humanity actually had begun to arrive a decade earlier when the railroads first entered the city, and even though Denver contained numerous hotels and facilities "for the protection and restoration of health," many of the newcomers, as well as large numbers of Denver businessmen, frequently left the city on temporary visits to nearby medicinal springs. To take advantage of this trend, Byer pre-empted the lands in nearby Middle Park known as Hot Sulphur Springs, built a crude cabin with an extended log roof projecting over the spring's principal basin, and began charging prospectors and tourists "six 'bits' for an entrance." Gradually a small town arose around the springs; in 1879, Frank Fossett noted that the site was "getting to be more and more a great resort."[11]

In his dual role as the editor of the *News* and as the proprietor

[10] Bickham, *From Ohio to the Rocky Mountains,* 69; H. H. Bancroft, *History of Nevada, Colorado, and Wyoming,* 374.

[11] Fossett, *Colorado: Its Gold and Silver Mines,* 96; Ernest Ingersoll, *Knocking Round the Rockies,* 55–56. Estes Park and Idaho Springs also were favorite nearby refuges for invalids and tired businessmen. Bickham, *From Ohio to the Rocky Mountains,* 159.

of a health resort, Byer became one of the most important boosters of northeastern Colorado. Proof of his effectiveness in this regard is the fact that the Territorial Board of Immigration and later the State Board of Health, both of which were actively engaged in advertising the state's health attractions as a whole, often called upon him for general and statistical information on the Denver area.[12]

Railroads quickly recognized the business value of advertising the health centers along their service routes, and the Union Pacific was particularly praiseworthy of Denver, the city it considered most "representative of the proportion of invalid and healthy residents of the State." In a most unusual format—by using the official mortuary reports for the years 1885–87—the railroad proved incontrovertibly that consumption was exceedingly rare among the residents of Denver and that only a few more than two hundred of the thousands of phthisical patients who came there annually actually died from the disease. Then, by quoting extensively from a paper written by Dr. Charles Denison, "the highest authority on the treatment of consumption in the high altitudes of Colorado," the Union Pacific offered prospective clients a real service by detailing the best method of obtaining maximum benefit from residency in the state. Short promotional resumés of four mineral spring resorts near Denver were also given.[13]

By 1890, Denver ranked with Colorado Springs as a favorite place among invalids and the vacationing public, even though a fair comparison of the two cities was hardly possible. Colorado Springs was first and foremost a health and pleasure resort, and

[12] See his contributions to: Colorado Territorial Board of Immigration, *Resources and Advantages of Colorado,* 10; Horn, "Report on the Mineral Springs of Colorado," *Annual Report,* (1877), 56–58.

[13] Union Pacific Railway Company, *Colorado: A Complete and Comprehensive Description,* 117–19, 120–24, 132–38. Another railroad with lands for sale in the Denver area also used the prospects of good health as a promotional "come-on." Chicago, Burlington and Quincy Railroad Co., *Eastern Colorado,* 7.

its principal attraction resulted from a near-holiday-type atmosphere. Denver, on the other hand, was the political and business center of the state, and as such it had a more practical appeal. For the well to do, the latter city offered better investment opportunities, a social life predominantly eastern in character, and diversionary activities suited to the most cultivated taste. Its famed Denver Club left any visitor "little to criticize," and touring artists, such as the world-famous Paderewski, often played to overflowing audiences in the city's best theaters. For those "who had to earn their own support" while convalescing, Denver afforded many employment opportunities and a reasonable cost of living. But for all, regardless of station, the best in medical attention was always available, since the city was the home of many well-trained physicians (including Denison and Fisk) and the site of several hospitals operated especially for consumptive patients.[14]

Colorado Springs and Samuel Edwin Solly were inseparable names in the late nineteenth century; the town became world famous because the doctor, who had recovered his health there, gratefully and masterfully promoted it as a health resort for consumptives. But the development of the city had its beginning in the mind of General William J. Palmer in 1870, four years before Solly arrived on the scene. While making route surveys for the Kansas Pacific Railway in 1868–69, Palmer became familiar with and impressed by the medicinal properties of the Iron, Soda, and Manitou springs near Pikes Peak and Ute Pass, and he foresaw the day when these springs would become a favorite gathering place for the health- and pleasure-seeking classes.

Unable, however, to persuade the Kansas Pacific to accept

[14] Lewis Morris Iddings, "Life in the Altitudes: Colorado's Health Plateau," *Scribner's Magazine,* Vol. XIX (February, 1896), 150; Fisk, "Colorado for Invalids," *Popular Science Monthly,* Vol. XXV (July, 1884), 315. For an early listing of Denver's tubercular hospitals, see Francis S. Kinder, "The Consumptive's Chances in Colorado," *Review of Reviews* (New York), Vol. XXVII (June, 1903), 698–702.

any of the route proposals arising from his surveys, he resigned in 1870 as the railroad's managing director, formed the Denver and Rio Grande Railway Company, along with William A. Bell and others, and embarked immediately upon the task of building a trunk line stretching southward from Denver along the base of the Rocky Mountains. Through a subsidiary organization of the new company, Palmer acquired ownership of Soda Springs and also of ten thousand acres of land at the base of Pikes Peak on which to build the rail center for the region. Colorado Springs was born on July 31, 1871, when the first stake was driven.

The town and its adjacent springs enjoyed a phenomenal growth—much faster, in fact, than its founders had anticipated. At the end of its first year of existence, 277 town lots had been sold, 159 houses were erected, and Colorado Springs boasted eight hundred permanent residents. In addition, a hotel was built at the springs, and a small village, first called La Font but later Manitou, began slowly to emerge.[15]

Resort facilities multiplied at such a pace that by 1876 Frank Fossett felt justified in calling Colorado Springs and Manitou Springs the "Saratoga of the West," and noted further that the cities had "a number of first class hotels that afford every accommodation known to eastern houses. Thousands of tourists and invalids," he concluded, "visit these beautiful towns annually to partake of the health giving water of Manitou, and to breathe that inspiring air that only Colorado can furnish." These "thousands" in the yearly tourist and invalid entourage reached thirty thousand by 1880 and two hundred thousand by 1890, a remarkable growth indeed for the development's short nineteen years' existence.[16]

[15] H. H. Bancroft, *History of Nevada, Colorado, and Wyoming,* 601 n., 603–604n.; Teetor, "Manitou Springs, All the Year Round," *Magazine of Western History,* Vol. XI (November, 1889), 46.

[16] Fossett, *Colorado: A Historical, Descriptive, and Statistical Work,* 452; Fossett, *Colorado: Its Gold and Silver Mines,* 38; Teetor, "Letter from Manitou Spring," *Magazine of Western History,* Vol. XIII (February, 1891), 435.

Such a growth could result only from sustained promotional efforts—these Colorado Springs got from many sources. Easily the most effective booster of the area's climate and mineral springs was Dr. Samuel Solly. So convincing were his professional articles that many of his eastern colleagues sent their consumptive patients to Colorado Springs without ever having visited the city. Equally persuasive on the public as a whole were his two reasonably comprehensive but highly readable pamphlets, the first issued in 1875 and the second in 1883, which gave meaningful analyses of the healing properties of the climate and waters at both Colorado Springs and Manitou Springs.[17] Solly loved these beautiful health centers and for the most part took an unselfish attitude in wanting to share their blessings with those who were bowed by disease.

The Denver and Rio Grande Railway also praised these resort centers but perhaps for more mundane reasons. Longer passenger lists meant greater profits from the use of company-owned rail and resort facilities. In an 1881 travel guide to *Health, Wealth and Pleasure in Colorado and New Mexico*, the Colorado Springs–Manitou area was described as "the most romantic and renowned watering-place of the Rocky Mountains and the tourist center of Colorado," and special tourist tickets were promised to all points of interest thereabouts which were serviced by the Denver and Rio Grande. Then, just two years later, General Palmer, seeking to capitalize upon the traffic his company's promotional literature helped to increase, opened the ostentatious Antlers Hotel, first of the truly great hotel resorts in Colorado.[18]

Unsolicited testimonials concerning the region's curative pow-

[17] *Manitou, Colorado, U.S.A., Its Mineral Waters and Climate;* Samuel Edwin Solly and Mrs. Simeon J. Dunbar, *The Health Resorts of Colorado Springs and Manitou.*

[18] Pueblo and Cañon City, two moderately popular resort centers, were among those serviced by the Denver and Rio Grande. Denver and Rio Grande Railway, *Health, Wealth and Pleasure in Colorado and New Mexico,* 22–38, 46; Pomeroy, *In Search of the Golden West,* 20.

ers and excellent accommodations came from almost every quarter during the eighties and nineties. "Of course we went to Manitou," A. A. Hayes, Jr., wrote in 1880, "for everyone goes thither. It is called the 'Saratoga of the West'—an appellation which pleases Manitou and does not harm Saratoga." And Hayes continued:

> . . . one may see men and women walking about, and using and enjoying life who long ago, if they had staid [*sic*] in the East, would have in Western parlance, "gone over the range . . . ." "Why, they keep me here for an example of the effects of the climate," said a worthy and busy man at Colorado Springs. "I came here from Chicago on a mattress." And so did many others.[19]

Dr. Charles Denison in the same year noted: "These springs, with their picturesque surroundings and tonic atmosphere, yearly attract many invalids to Manitou, which is rapidly gaining favor, both as a summer and winter resort." His Denver colleague, Dr. Samuel Fisk, commented in 1884 that "Colorado Springs combines so many favorable conditions of climate, good accommodations, pleasant society, and natural objects of interest, as to render it . . . an almost ideal resort for phthisical invalids." Ernest Ingersoll after a summer's ramble in the Rockies in 1885 added elaborate appraisals of the hostelries of the "mountain spa," of the therapeutic qualities of the waters, and of many desirable excursions which were available to Manitou tourists. Louis R. Ehrich, a New York City merchant who recovered from tuberculosis at the Springs in 1887 and who later became a stockholder in the Manitou Mineral Water Company, wrote that had he known of Colorado Springs earlier he could "have saved over five years of fruitless wandering in Europe and would today be far richer in health and richer in purse." And Henry Dudley Teetor, a feature writer for the *Magazine of Western History*

19 "Vacation Aspects of Colorado," *Harper's New Monthly Magazine*, Vol. LX (March, 1880), 544–45.

and a frequent guest at Manitou's society-conscious Cliff House, always entranced his readers with descriptions of the cultural life and health-restoring atmosphere at the springs.[20]

Perhaps Lewis Iddings in 1896 summed up most adequately the results of Colorado Springs's first twenty-five years of development by stating that he, in common with most observers, thought the resort easily led all others in the Rocky Mountains in "answering most requirements" of sick people who "must confine themselves most of the time in places where there are good hotels, or boarding-houses, or comfortable houses to rent." And he also was cognizant of the great contribution which the health trade had made to the economy of the town:

> The value of the invalid population to the town is pretty generally understood by the authorities . . . . A prominent banker estimates that the invalid community, apart from those engaged in trade, spends over half a million a year. This expenditure helped to keep Colorado Springs from greatly feeling the hard times which oppressed the country in 1893–94. Not a bank failed; the business remained in excellent shape; rents did not come down materially, and the town went through the panic years without much danger.[21]

In a single generation, energetic promoters, in partnership with a benevolent nature, raised Colorado Springs to the top of the better-known, more fashionable Rocky Mountain oases.

Resort centers along the foothills and plains of eastern Colorado

20 Denison, *Rocky Mountain Health Resorts*, 40; Fisk, "Colorado for Invalids," *Popular Science Monthly*, Vol. XXV (July, 1884), 315; Ingersoll, *Crest of the Continent*, 36–40. The published accounts of Ehrich's personal experiences, printed first in the New York *Tribune* (May 22, 1887) and later in pamphlet form, were remarkable pieces of promotional literature. See Louis R. Ehrich, *Health Resorts for Lung Troubles*. Ehrich's company, the Manitou Mineral Water Company, by 1891 was shipping two million bottles of water into all parts of the United States. Teetor, "Letter from Manitou Springs," *Magazine of Western History*, Vol. V (1888), 436; Teetor, "Manitou Springs, All the Year Round," *ibid.*, Vol. XI (November, 1889), 43–47.

21 "Life in the Altitudes: Colorado's Health Plateau," *Scribner's Magazine*, Vol. XIX (February, 1896), 39, 147–48.

enjoyed the decisive advantage of accessibility, and this fact explains, for the most part, why their growth was both early and phenomenal. A majority of the mineral springs in central and western Colorado, though long known, could not be reached by rail until the early eighties, and some of them not until the early nineties.[22] Consequently, their growth was gradual and their promotion sporadic until adequate transportation service was made available.

The more remote watering places received their first serious promotion by Dr. T. G. Horn in 1877 and 1878. After appointment to the State Board of Health for Colorado, Horn conducted a two-year survey of the mineral springs in the state and published his findings in the first two issues of the board's annual reports.[23] This synthesis, which he considered imperfect because of the absence of adequate published materials on many of the springs, was nonetheless quite revealing; the state abounded with mineral springs of the types known to be "most beneficial" to humanity, and some of them already were in advanced stages of development. Three near Denver—Hot Sulphur Springs, Morrison Springs, and Idaho Springs—boasted "first class" hotels.

Of the three, Idaho Springs was regarded as the most promisingly located and ideally endowed, but by 1889 a yearly average of only five hundred patrons were "entertained" during the summer months at the town's three hotels and "several boarding houses." Still, those who resorted there were highly complimentary of the place. Henry Dudley Teetor, a guest for a night at

22 This was not true of those in southern Colorado. The Denver and Rio Grande, in a magnificent engineering feat, crossed Vita Pass in 1878 and brought most of the springs in that area within reach of all classes of visitors. H. H. Bancroft, *History of Nevada, Colorado, and Wyoming*, 554.

23 Horn, "Report on the Mineral Springs of Colorado," *First Annual Report* of the Secretary of the State Board of Health of the State of Colorado (1877), 47–65; "Report on the Mineral Springs of Colorado," *Second Annual Report* of the State Board of Health of Colorado (1878), 43–55. For one person's impression of these reports see Teetor, "Some of the Mineral Springs of Colorado," *Magazine of Western History*, Vol. XIII (January, 1891), 304–307.

the Hotel Stanton in 1890, rested in deep, "dreamless sleep" and arose to find a most agreeable "sun-bright clime" and a charming community of friendly, healthy people.[24]

The slow progress of Idaho Springs was characteristic of all "would-be Saratogas" in central and western Colorado and symptomatic of the over-all trend in western excursion traffic. Invalids and tourists enjoyed the pioneering thrills that came with thumping down steep mountain grades along narrow-gauge rails, but a vast majority of these travelers sought a more refined and festive environment—for them a visit of two or three days at one of the more remote Colorado watering places was sufficient.[25] The principal urge was for southern California. Even the popular "promoted tours," which were arranged in eastern cities by such travel agencies as Raymond and Whitcomb of Boston, allowed their vacation-minded clientele no more than a few hours for side trips while whisking them along the transcontinental lines to vacations on the sun-drenched beaches of the Pacific Ocean.

The most frequently patronized of these stopover health resorts was Glenwood Springs in western Colorado. When the Denver and Rio Grande Railway finally reached Glenwood in 1887, only modest accommodations were available for tired and delicate travelers, but with the completion of the five-story Hotel Colorado in 1893, the city (and western Colorado) had its first great resort hotel. Thereafter, visitors were "enraptured with the mere view of the place." Glenwood was "covered by nothing but the blue sky, and surrounded or enclosed only by Dame Nature's breath—the atmosphere"; the resort's man-made bathing pool, supplied with free-flowing 127 degree mineralized water, was so big (six hundred feet in length) that all "other fashionable pools seem baby-like by comparison"; and the grand Hotel Colorado

[24] "One Summer Day at Idaho Springs," *ibid.*, Vol. XIII (November, 1890), 15–19; Denison, "The Mineral Springs of Colorado," *Transactions of the American Climatological Association*, Vol. VI (1889), 222–223.

[25] Pomeroy, *In Search of the Golden West*, 22.

was "as fine in every detail as any hotel at any pleasure or health resort in the East." Despite its beautiful setting and excellent facilities, Glenwood's patrons generally passed only "a few days there rather than a season," and the incoming volume was never comparable to that at Manitou Springs.[26]

A fabulous hotel and bubbling hot springs were the chief factors in making Las Vegas Hot Springs, New Mexico, a considerable resort for health- and pleasure-seekers in the late nineteenth century. Located just six miles northwest of Old Las Vegas, a landmark on the Santa Fe Trail, these springs had been used for medicinal purposes by Indians, Spaniards, fur trappers, and Santa Fe tradesmen for a period spanning several centuries. But apparently the United States Army made the first serious improvements at the springs in 1846 when it erected an adobe bathhouse and a hospital on the site for use by diseased and wounded soldiers of the Mexican War. These buildings, later abandoned by the army during the Civil War, were the only accommodations available to resorters until 1879.

With that date, the history of the fabled *Los Ojos Calientes* as a health resort began; it was then that W. S. Moore bought the property, started construction of the Hot Springs Adobe Hotel, and became "a one man Chamber of Commerce to make the nation Hot Springs conscious."[27] When the Atchison, Topeka and Santa Fe Railway reached nearby Las Vegas, Moore created such interest among its officials that they not only built a six mile spur line to the springs but a year later bought out Moore's interest in the property completely.

Promotion of and construction at the springs mushroomed.

[26] Henry D. Schroeder, "A Study of the Highly Mineralized Thermal Waters . . . at the Glenwood Hot Springs, Colorado," *Transactions of the American Climatological Association*, Vol. XII (1896), 225–45; Julian Ralph, "Colorado's Unique Resort," *Harper's Weekly Magazine*, Vol. XXXVIII (March 17, 1894), 253; Pomeroy, *In Search of the Golden West*, 23.

[27] One of Moore's earliest patrons was Jesse James of Missouri, although it was "not generally known." Stanley, *The Las Vegas Story*, 293.

Advertised as a "delightful half-way resting place on the way to the Pacific," the Santa Fe announced that all through-passengers who held first-class tickets would be allowed "stop-over privileges" at the springs.[28] Then on April 17, 1882, the company opened the Montezuma Hotel, a magnificent Queen Anne type of structure costing $200,000. The 270-room hotel enjoyed a remarkable, if brief, success; it was frequently filled to capacity with well-bred patrons, and its adjoining bathhouse, which accommodated five hundred bathers, was often overcrowded. Then tragedy struck. In the wintry night hours of January 18, 1884, the Montezuma was destroyed by an uncontrollable fire, the nemesis of several of the early resort hotels.[29]

Patiently, the Santa Fe constructed a new and allegedly fireproof hotel, appropriately called the Phoenix, on a site "higher up on the hill-side."[30] For a time, much of the old grandeur was recaptured, but by the early nineties the heyday of Las Vegas had passed; its once heavy, but obviously fickle, tourist trade began to seek more fashionable pastures. The hotel register which once "read like an international 'Who's Who' " gradually became filled with less prominent names and, then, precious few names at all. Shortly after the turn of the century, the registry was closed forever; the mighty Montezuma (Phoenix) was closed and later sold by its owners to the Las Vegas YMCA for one dollar.[31]

[28] See the Atchison, Topeka and Santa Fe Railway advertisement, inside back cover, in George A. Crofutt, *Crofutt's Grip-Sack Guide to Colorado: A Complete Encyclopedia of the State.*

[29] *Las Vegas Hot Springs,* 5–6, 12. The Hotel Raymond in Pasedena and the Cliff House in San Francisco were destroyed by fire around the turn of the century. See pictures and comments in the front of Pomeroy, *In Search of the Golden West.*

[30] The name "Phoenix" was never popular; patrons persisted in calling the new structure the "Montezuma." Atchison, Topeka and Santa Fe Railway Co., *Las Vegas Hot Springs, New Mexico,* 11.

[31] Quoted from the diary of William Prager, thirty years a watchman at the Springs, in Stanley, *The Las Vegas Story,* 304–305. Since 1937, the Montezuma has been operated by Jesuits as a seminary "for the training of Mexican youth to serve as priests in their homeland." Lynn I. Perrigo, *Historic Sites in and near the "Meadow City."*

The early success of Las Vegas caused considerable excitement in New Mexican communities possessing similar medicinal springs, and by 1885, Ojo Caliente Springs in Taos County, Jemez Hot Springs in Bernalillo County, and Hudson Hot Springs in Grant County offered hotels and bathhouses to the resort-minded public.[32] Realizing their magnetic appeal to potential tourists and residents, the Territory's Bureau of Immigration gave these and lesser springs considerable space in its promotional literature. One pamphlet, issued in 1898, was unique; mixing solicited testimonials and scientific water analyses, the bureau listed every mineral and thermal spring in New Mexico and gave a short summary of the accommodations (if any) available at each. Typical of the private appraisals from prominent health-seekers was one contributed by A. G. Spalding, a wealthy Chicago sporting goods manufacturer:

> To whom it may concern: This is to say that I have visited Hudson Hot Springs . . . several times during the past six years. . . . I believe that the mineral waters of these hot springs are equal, if not superior, to any in America, for the cure of rheumatism, kidney and blood diseases, as well as indigestion and stomach disorders. . . . I believe, also that the climate at Hudson is the best and most equable all the year round to be found in the United States.[33]

Encouraging though such praise was, it helped none of the smaller springs reach even the shadow of Las Vegas' stature.

Santa Fe enjoyed a moderate reputation as a resort center, and consumptives particularly found its climate inviting. But even as late as 1896 the city still lacked the hotel accommodations necessary to make it a resort of the first rank.[34] This was true also of Albuquerque and other smaller New Mexican towns which

[32] Ritch, *New Mexico, Historical and Industrial,* 73–77.

[33] New Mexico Territorial Bureau of Immigration, *Bulletin No. 1, New Mexico, 1898: Climate, Mineral Springs, Schools,* 19.

[34] Iddings, "Life in the Altitudes: Colorado's Health Plateau," *Scribner's Magazine,* Vol. XIX (February, 1896), 139.

had nothing but a salubrious climate with which to attract tourists and invalids.

One characteristic of the invalid traffic in Texas and Arizona in the late nineteenth century is quite obvious—much of it was composed of indigents or of people of fairly modest means. Proof of this fact rests in the absence of great resort hotels in the Montezuma class. Although thousands poured into both regions every year, the demand for fashionable quarters was never great enough to encourage the investment necessary to build such establishments, and consumptive convalescents, regardless of financial status, were obliged either to accept whatever facilities were available to the general traveler or to improvise such accommodations as were needed or could be afforded. A sizeable number of destitute invalids lived in isolated tent cities or hired out as ranch hands; an even larger number lived in marginal quarters in towns where they could find enough part-time work to tide them over until improved health would permit more strenuous pursuits. Yet there was no hard and fast rule on where a particular class of health-seeker might be found; even a man of substantial means was frequently found beneath a canvas top or astride a quarter horse.

That such southwestern cities as San Antonio, El Paso, Tucson, and Phoenix became favorite "resting places" for thousands of tuberculars is well confirmed, but each did so with a minimum of promotion and with only a small number of resort facilities. Boosters might in all honesty depict San Antonio as "the most famous health resort in America," yet the city offered but one center of any size designed especially to cater to the needs of invalids, the modest eighty-room Hot Sulphur Wells Hotel and its adjacent bathhouse with a capacity of forty-five persons.[35] A few of the smaller resort towns and mineral springs in the vicin-

[35] These structures did not appear until the late nineties and were never widely advertised. *The City of San Antonio, Texas,* 2, 8–9; *Opportunities for the Homeseeker: Texas, The Coming Country, The Newest Southwest,* 8, 37–38.

ity of San Antonio had facilities equal to if not greater than those at the Hot Sulphur Wells.[36] Similarly, invalids who were attracted to Tucson by the "assiduous promotion" of such men as Patrick Hamilton, usually found quarters available only with other lungers in the endless rows of white tents which stretched from the city limits almost to the foothills of the nearby Catalina Mountains. Conditions in El Paso and Phoenix were not much better.[37]

After the turn of the century, Mineral Wells, Texas, enjoyed a phenomenal growth and made a bid for national acclaim as "the coming Carlsbad of America." Mineral waters, with varying contents, eventually were drawn from over four hundred wells, including the famed Crazy Well which was discovered in 1885, and by 1910, over 150,000 patrons thronged annually into the city's many hotels and bathhouses in order to drink of or bathe in Nature's miracle waters. By 1920, Mineral Wells was regarded as a major resort city as well as a favorite convention town for clubs and associations of all types. A smaller complex of hot (147 degrees), subsurface mineral waters was discovered in the early nineties at Marlin, Texas, and that city also thereafter enjoyed a substantial health trade. But despite the fact that Marlin offered adequate lodgings, a trained medical faculty, and an invitingly healthful environment, its development never reached Mineral Wells's dimensions.[38]

36 Boerne and Luling Springs offered a modest selection of accommodations. Durand, *San Antonio, Texas: The City of Missions,* 66; Galveston, Harrisburg and San Antonio Railway, *Western Texas as a Winter Resort: via the "Sunset Route,"* 29–31.

37 Patrick Hamilton, *The Resources of Arizona,* 130–42; Dean [William Richard] Harris, *By Path and Trail,* 205; *El Paso, Texas: A Story of Sunshine,* 1, 13; Craig, "Climatography of Arizona, with Especial Reference to the Climatic Treatment of Pulmonary Tuberculosis," *Journal of the American Medical Association,* Vol. XXXIX (October 4, 1902), 230.

38 "Texas' Carlsbad," *The Texas and Pacific Quarterly,* Vol. VIII (July, 1905), 27–31; *Texas Almanac [for 1910] and State Industrial Guide,* 325; W. P. Webb, *Handbook of Texas,* II, 213; Thomas Turner, "Eager Empire," *Texas Parade,* Vol. XX (April, 1960), 30–31. Wooten Wells, a nearby mineral-water resort, suffered a drastic loss of patrons when the Marlin wells were developed after 1892. Patrons eventually disappeared entirely. The chief cause was a matter of simple

Although a considerable number of free-spending pleasure-seekers frequented these resorts which were late in developing, both Mineral Wells and Marlin managed to resist the urge to cater only to that class of tourist. Both continued well into the twentieth century to offer moderately priced accommodations to health-seekers and vacationers alike. This was not true of many of the older resort centers. More and more crowded by the elite of the nation's tourists, the "better" resorts became increasingly expensive—almost prohibitively so for many money-conscious invalids. About the inflated economy of one watering place, Lewis Iddings wrote:

> Colorado Springs is not a cheap place. The Antlers is an acceptable hotel, constantly improving but expensive. . . . Rent houses strike a newcomer as appalling—$250 to $350 a month is pretty steep, even for a well-furnished, commodious house, but people pay these rents calmly after a preliminary grumbling and last winter, despite the hard times, desirable furnished dwellings were hard to find.[39]

The high cost of health-seeking in the late 1890's so moved one invalid doctor that he set for himself the task

> . . . contingent, of course, upon my own recovery . . . to bring the cost of coming West for health's sake . . . within the means of people of moderate financial resources, and, of course, to supply them with just as good care, food and treatment as could be obtained at home.[40]

This humble humanitarian, Dr. E. S. Bullock, built and became

preference; Marlin's warm waters were far more desirable than those at Wooten Wells which were so cold that they had to "cool" after being drawn from eighty-foot wells before patients could bathe in them comfortably. Turner, "Early Health Resort Lives Only in Memory," Dallas *Morning News,* February 17, 1948.

39 "Life in the Altitudes: Colorado's Health Plateau," *Scribner's Magazine,* Vol. XIX (February, 1896), 147. Dr. Samuel Fisk also cautioned that where money, and not health and comfort, was a prime concern, invalids ought to consider some place other than Colorado Springs. Fisk, "Colorado for Invalids," *Popular Science Monthly,* Vol. XXV (July, 1884), 315.

40 E. S. Bullock, "The Southwest as a Resort for Pulmonary Patients," *Journal of the Outdoor Life,* Vol. III (1906–1907), 47.

the medical director of the New Mexico Cottage Sanatorium at Silver City, the first low-budget sanatorium of its type in the Southwest. Yet the hospital's original capacity (twenty patients) was so small that its influence was not felt immediately.

Economic considerations exerted a great influence on the patterns of invalid migration, but a more powerful determinant in the late nineteenth century was the growing realization that phthisis was a contagious disease and that resorts were potential centers for its dissemination. "It is a noticeable fact," Dr. Frederick J. Bancroft wrote in 1889, "that the health-resorts in America have, after a time, lost much of their reputation for the relief of phthisis."[41] Recognizing their patrons' deep concern in this regard, managers of the better hotels at first posted signs which read, "Guests will please take their medicines in their rooms," and ultimately refused (and so advertised) to admit consumptives. Dr. C. H. Alden commented on the trend in California thusly:

> The attitude of Southern Californians toward incoming tuberculous invalids has undergone a change during the past few years. Formerly such invalids brought in needed money and were freely welcome, but . . . [it] is now becoming difficult for consumptives to obtain suitable accommodations in hotels and boarding houses, or by renting.[42]

Francis Kinder met with similar resistance at Denver:

> . . . some time ago [I] had the care of a brother with lung trouble, and being in need of larger quarters, rented a house. The landlord, after receiving the rent, asked about sickness, and on being told the facts he returned the rent, declaring that his tenants in the neighborhood would leave were a consumptive so near.[43]

41 "About Health Resorts," *Magazine of Western History*, Vol. XI (December, 1889), 171.

42 "Some Southern California Health Resorts," *Transactions of the American Climatological Association*, Vol. XXI (1905), 46.

43 "The Consumptive's Chances in Colorado," *Review of Reviews* (New York), Vol. XXVII (June, 1903), 698.

Thus, great changes were in the making by the turn of the century. Once dependent upon an invalid trade, many resort hotels and centers became openly (and ungratefully) hostile to the health-seeker and almost indifferent to his pressing needs for comfortable accommodations and expert medical attention. Koch's tiny bacillus had cast a Gargantuan shadow of fear over the southwestern health frontier, forcing a reappraisal of resort centers, climate, mineral waters, and even the poor lunger.

VIII. *The Death of a Legend: Reappraisal and Readjustment*

Around the turn of the century, a tiny parasitic bacillus destroyed almost as many myths as it did people. Time-honored theories of disease contagion and patiently developed techniques in medical and climatic therapeutics were practically revolutionized when it was discovered that consumption is a communicable disease, carried in a highly infectious stage by the afflicted and disseminated among the unsuspecting through personal contact or poor sanitary habits. Unfortunately, Koch's brilliant discovery was not followed by an immediate assurance of the control or cure of tuberculosis. For an indefinite period the disease continued to threaten everyone with its insidious contamination and to inflict death upon a frightening percentage of its victims. The resulting "phthisiophobia" wrought significant changes not only in medical practices but in the whole concept of a frontier for health.

In the matter of treatment, consumption had always been "a disease of fads"; an imperfect understanding of causal factors had narrowed the physician's activities to the field of therapy, and a variety of hopeful panaceas were introduced in an effort to control the disease. "A man need not be old in the medical profession," Dr. Mark Rodgers wrote in 1906,

> to remember the treatment of pulmonary tuberculosis by rectal injections of sulphuretted hydrogen gas; the treatment by Koch's lymph; the climatic treatment; creosote, guiacol, cod-liver oil, X-Ray, Christian science, osteopathy and what-not.[1]

None of these remedial agents had proved effective in checking the spread of tuberculosis, but the reasons for each failure became intelligible only after the tubercule bacillus had been isolated. Recognition of the new causal truth was universal if not instantaneous.

"Ten or twelve years ago," a deeply concerned Dr. William Russell admitted in 1897,

> even the most advanced physicians were not agreed that consumption belonged to the communicable diseases, and practically none took any steps to prevent its spread from the sick to the well. In fact, there were not a few who denied that it was ever contracted in this way. Heredity, physical conformation, atmospheric and soil conditions were regarded as the important factors, and all efforts were directed to the study and control of these. To-day there is an entire change of position. Communicability stands first in importance, and there are few who deny that it is the essential factor in the perpetuation of the disease.[2]

Old fads gave way to new ones. Prophylaxis (for the skilled practitioner) and hygiene (for the general public) rapidly became the accepted stratagems; "everybody," a 1901 appraisal of the new trend ran, "knows what microbes are, and can repeat the last warnings of hyper-careful physicians about [the] possibilities of infection."[3] And even though the disease continued to defy all medicines, decreasing attention was shown thereafter to such therapeutic practices as making hasty pilgrimages to dis-

[1] "Some Observations on Tuberculosis by a Dweller in the Desert," *Charities Review,* Vol. XVI (September 1, 1906), 558.

[2] "Consumption and Consumptives," *Popular Science Monthly,* Vol. L (January, 1897), 336.

[3] "The Search for Health," *Spectator,* Vol. LXXXVII (September 21, 1901), 382.

tant aseptic climates, drinking large volumes of highly mineralized waters, or avoiding contact with once feared fogs and miasmata.

The pulmonary invalid suffered immeasurably not only from the deadly bacillus but from a drastic shift in public sentiment. Once treated everywhere with humanitarian respect as the pitiable victim of an epidemic environment, he now was coldly rejected as the unwelcomed bearer of a lecherous bacteria. Subtlety was not a characteristic of this change in attitude. One author suggested that consumptives be made to wear bells around their necks to inform (or warn) others of their whereabouts; another insisted that rooms be disinfected and sleeping cars fumigated after their use by phthisics; still another warned that tuberculars must be prevented from spitting in public places since this was "the chief means of spreading infection."[4] Most damning of all, however, was the injurious, but medically feasible, comparison of the nineteenth-century lunger with the ancient leper, an analogy which found frequent expression among physicians who regarded complete isolation as the safest method of controlling both diseases.

Such a conclusion inherently identified the chief casualty in the transition to bacteriological science—climate no longer was considered the major factor in controlling tuberculosis. Though never totally discounted as a remedial agent, climate nonetheless came to be regarded as nothing better than a valuable adjuvant. Spokesmen for the new age of medicine denied that any climate had a specific curative quality and declared that all fresh air, regardless of location, possessed essentially the same attributes.[5]

[4] W. K. McClure, "Boycott of Consumptives," *The Living Age*, Vol. CCLI (December 8, 1906), 627n.; Benedict, "Consumption Considered as a Contagious Disease," *Popular Science Monthly*, Vol. XLVIII (November, 1895), 37, 39; George Holme, "A Mountain Home for Consumptives," *Munsey's Magazine*, Vol. XXVII (August, 1902), 757.

[5] S. A. Knopf, M.D., "The Tuberculosis Problem in the United States," *North American Review*, Vol. CXLVIII (February, 1899), 220.

Similar attacks were made on the use of thermal and mineral waters. Dr. Woods Hutchinson, a leader in debunking the excessive claims of resort proprietors, regarded the use of mineral waters as a potpourri of superstition, tradition, and ignorance. Most of the *au natural* waters, he asserted, could be reproduced at home from hydrant or well water at a fraction of the costs incurred in visiting a commercialized spa. He was, however, quick to recognize the real virtues in "taking the water cure":

> A three weeks' cure—which is the "standard" length the world over—means a three weeks' vacation in a delightful open-air resort, with plenty of people who are doing just exactly what you are, and are willing to listen to your symptoms on condition of being allowed to relate theirs in return.
>
> This is precisely the kind of company which an invalid really wants . . . he is utterly lost and out of place among vigorous healthy people . . . that have not time to sit and "swap symptoms" with him . . . he has "no one to play with."[6]

The sympathetic companionship found in such abundance at resort centers was, to Hutchinson, far more valuable as a therapeutic agent than "eight-tenths of the world's mineral waters," waters which he defined as being little more than "weak sea-water."

It was inevitable that professional attacks on climate and medicinal waters would eventually become directed toward the Southwest, for it was upon these two natural attributes that the region's reputation as a health frontier was based. It is important to note, however, that much of this criticism was leveled at a fleeting legend, not at an established dogma. The legend of perfect health in the Southwest was originally created by restored invalids and was later perpetuated by resort promoters; western physicians were not overly victimized by this loosely supported myth, for they knew from prolonged experience that the area's

[6] "Taking the Waters: The Humbug of Hot Springs," *Everybody's Magazine*, Vol. XXVIII (February, 1913), 162, 166.

climate was more of a "cure-some" than a "cure-all." Nor were these doctors attempting to be overly dogmatic when they referred to the Southwest as the healthiest section in the nation, for this distinction unquestionably was, and still is, accurate. Only a minor part of the criticism which follows was aimed at western climatologists, but even that small portion appears unwarranted in view of the facts.

Despite the absence of a serious inner-fraternal quarrel, the assault came and the legend fell with a resounding thud. Barely a year after the discovery of the bacillus, Frank Carpenter let loose a vitriolic denunciation of what he felt were the exaggerated claims of climatic benefits in the western country. "Never," he declared,

> was the evidence more one-sided than that upon the climate cure . . . . The friends of the Rocky Mountain region claim that the presence of consumption in their mortality-lists is due solely to the influx of invalids who are in a dying condition on their arrival, and beyond all hope of possible recovery; but it should be remembered that the resident population of this frontier is made up of robust pioneers and adventurers, of the toughest physical material, upon which, whether in Connecticut or in Colorado, consumption could make no impression.[7]

The obviously unreliable nature of such assertions, he said, was aggravated by the fact that none of the major witnesses—physicians, railway managers, hotel proprietors, real estate promoters, guidebook publishers, or even invalids themselves—could be considered unprejudiced authorities; each group had a service to sell or a reputation to uphold and was likely to view the "salutary qualities of the climate" with a biased eye. "Meanwhile," Carpenter retorted,

> the thousands who have died are lying silent in their graves, unable to add their testimony, and the hundreds who are dying are

[7] "The Climate Cure," *Lippincott's Magazine*, Vol. XXXI (April, 1883), 394.

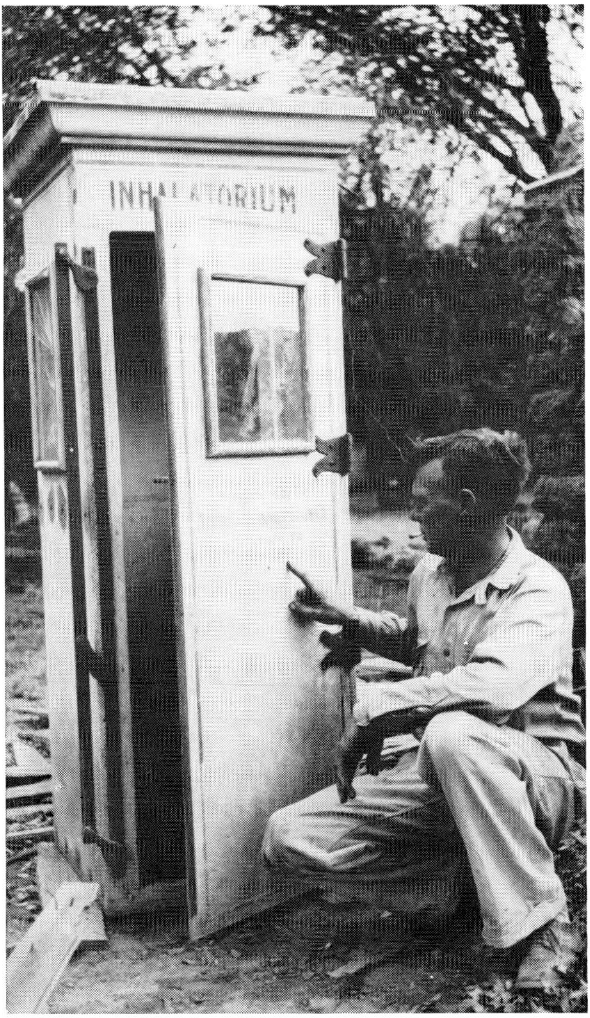

At Will Pruett's tent city near Fort Davis, Texas, this unique "Inhalatorium" was used by tuberculars to breathe medicinal vapors pumped into the closed chamber.

Photograph by Barry Scobee, Fort Davis, Texas

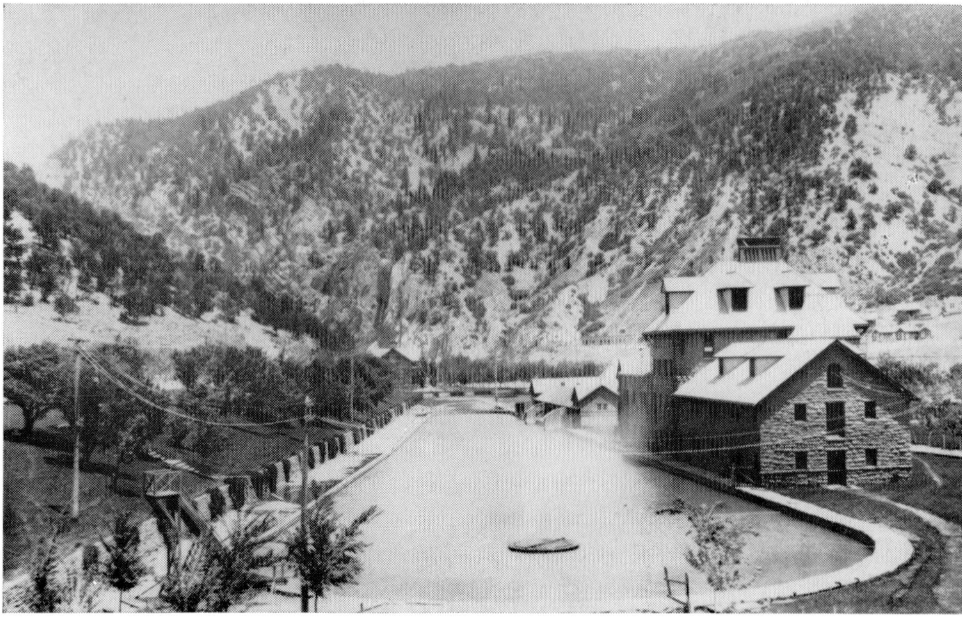

Today's visitors to Glenwood Springs, Colorado, will recognize this 600-foot-long pool, which made all other fashionable pools "seem baby-like by comparison." Here patients could take comfort from the 127-degree mineralized waters.

Photograph by Rose Hopkins,
courtesy Denver Public Library Western Collection

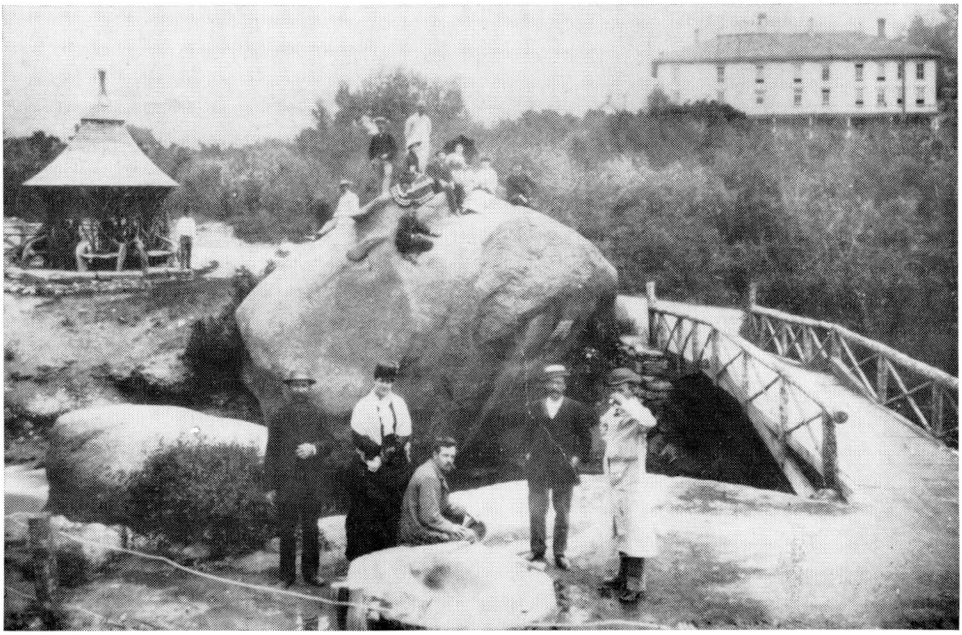

High in the mountains near Colorado Springs, Colorado, are the famous Manitou Soda Springs. In this photograph fashionable resorters are drinking the mineralized waters, thought to benefit internal afflictions.

Photograph by W. H. Jackson,
courtesy Denver Public Library Western Collection

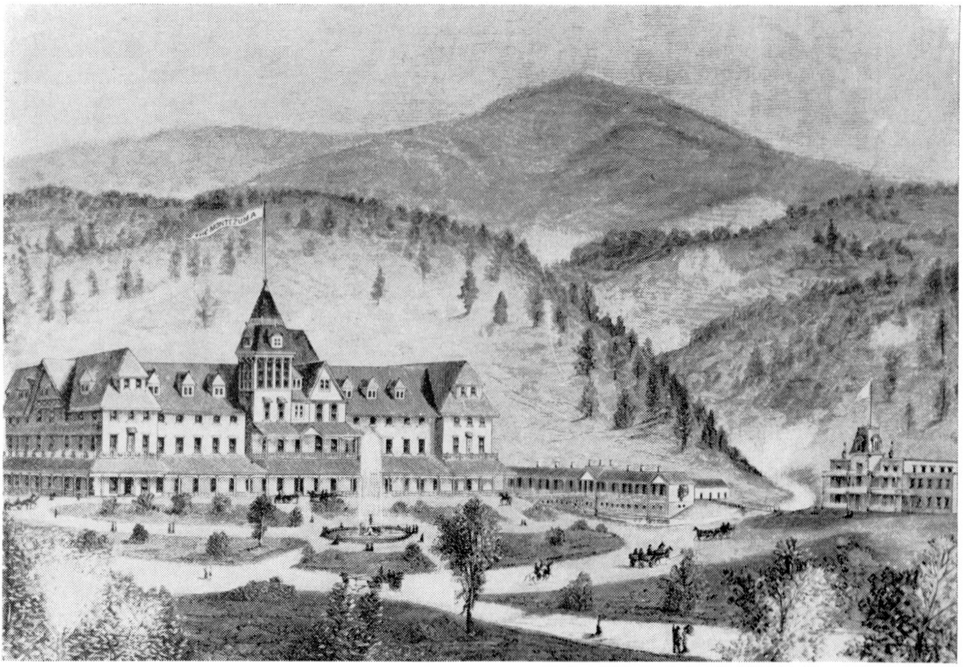

The mighty Montezuma was constructed in 1882 at Las Vegas Hot Springs, New Mexico, by the Atchison, Topeka and Santa Fe Railway to attract the more affluent health-seekers and excursionists.

Courtesy Denver Public Library Western Collection

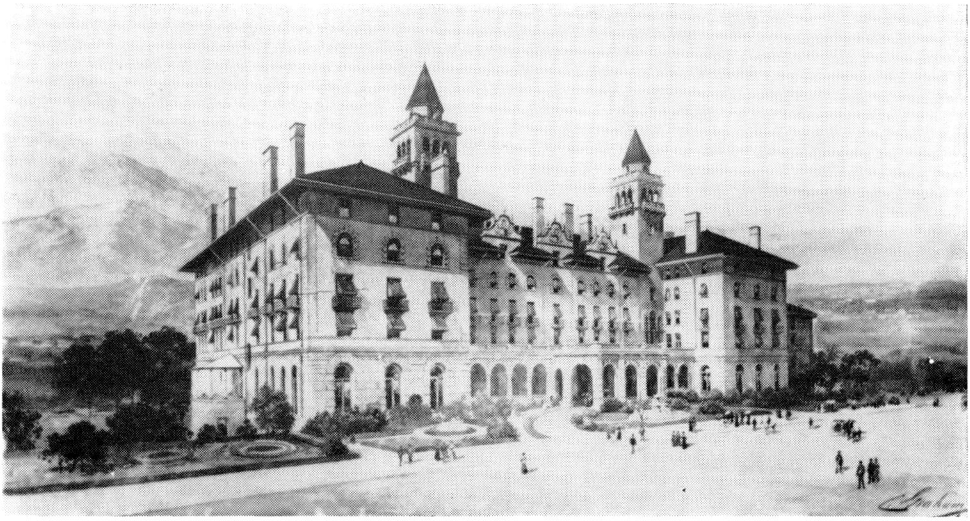

The Antlers Hotel, built at Colorado Springs in 1883 by the Denver and Rio Grande Railroad partly to cater to the western invalid traffic, has only recently been torn down.

Courtesy Denver Public Library Western Collection

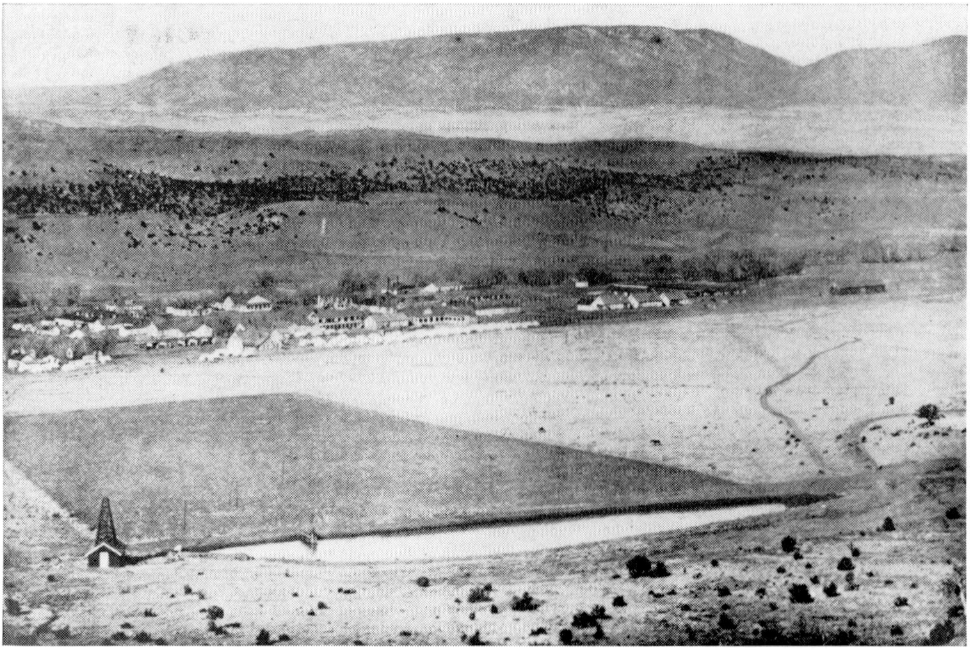

Fort Stanton, near Roswell, New Mexico, was established for use as a sanatorium for "seamen employed on vessels of the merchant marine . . . keepers and crews of lighthouses, officers and men of the Revenue Cutter Service and the Coast and Geodetic Survey, and officers and men employed on government vessels other than navy."

Courtesy Denver Public Library Western Collection

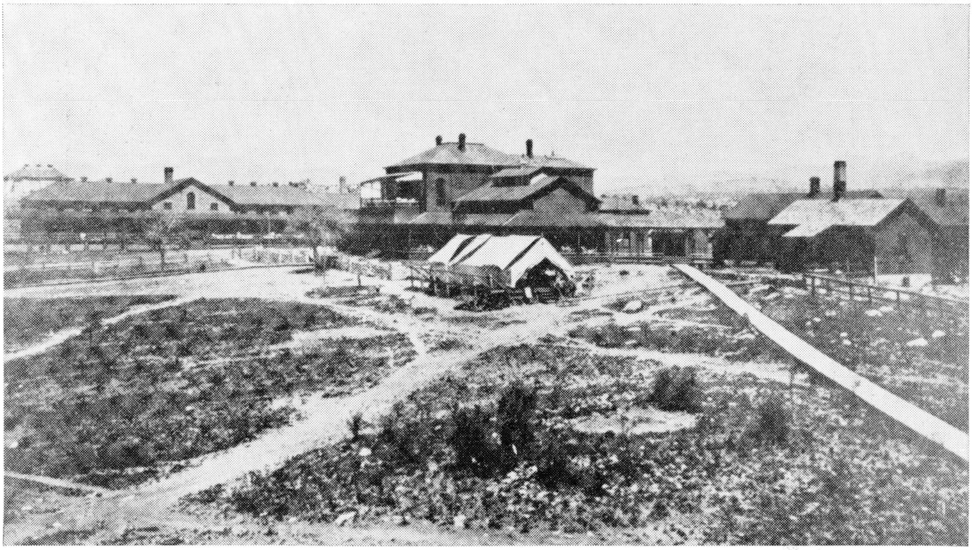

Fort Bayard, near Silver City, New Mexico, served "officers and men of the army and navy who . . . contracted tuberculosis in the government service."

Courtesy Denver Public Library Western Collection

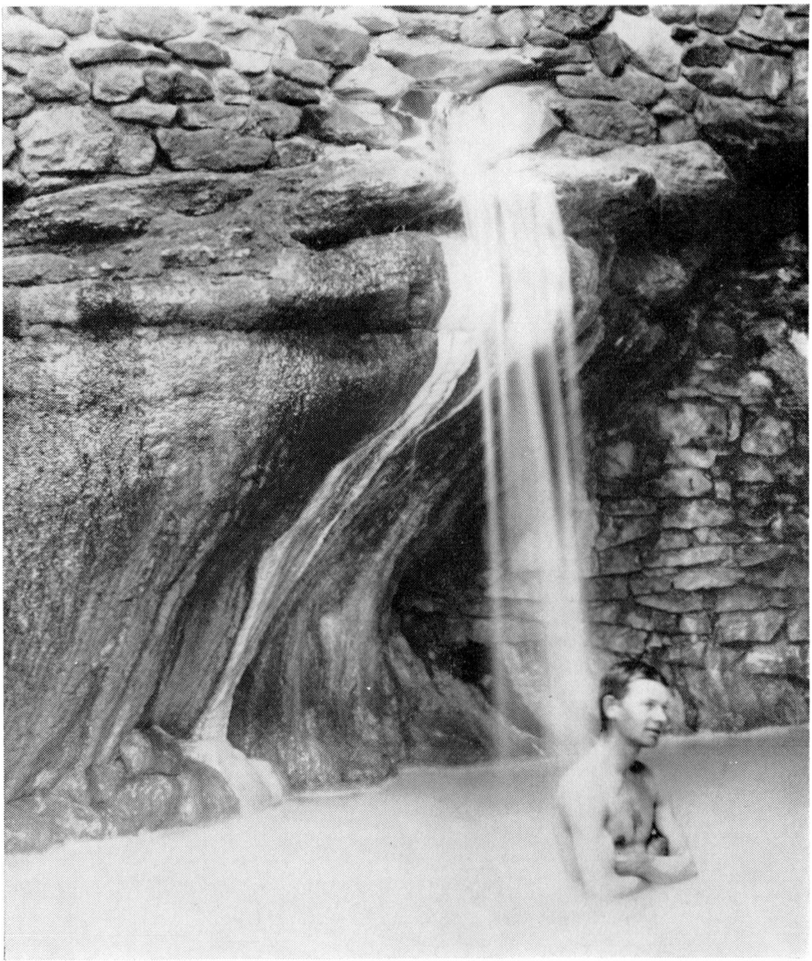

A bather soaks in the warm sulphurated waters of Hot Sulphur Springs, Colorado.

Courtesy Denver Public Library Western Collection

> unwilling to admit the gloomy fact, or are adverse to discussing a subject which cannot be otherwise than painful to them.

Actually, warnings to the effect that western climates were not always favorable came much earlier than Carpenter's depressing observations. Dr. Samuel Solly noted in 1880 that climate, like a two-edged sword, often cut both ways and was piercingly cruel to those who misused it. Winslow Ayer observed in the same year that "it is true that very many have found death, when they had confidently hoped for new life," but, he concluded, "it is seldom that a timely and sufficiently protracted visit is not attended with signal benefit, if not indeed entire restoration."[8]

Later alarms were sounded from all quarters. Dr. Samuel Fisk, after observing one hundred cases of tuberculosis over a two-year period, was shocked to learn that less than 50 per cent were still living at the time of his final tabulation, a figure hardly complimentary of Colorado's climate. Dr. Thomas Darlington, a resident physician at Bisbee, Arizona, who was dubious of hot, dry climates in treating diseases, reported in 1891 that out of a controlled group of fifty-eight persons under his observation, only one had shown any improvement from a residence in the territory. Dr. H. G. Wetherill, a New Jersey consumptive who toured most of the major resort areas of the Southwest in 1892–93, found western climates supported by so many fallacies that he felt duty bound to warn his eastern colleagues "to exercise rare good judgement" in selecting patients to be sent to the region.[9] In 1894, Colorado's State Board of Health departed sharply from a previously held claim that consumption was almost unknown among

[8] Solly, quoted in Hayes, *New Colorado and the Santa Fe Trail,* 184; Ayer, *Life in the Wilds of America,* 232.

[9] Fisk, "Further Considerations of the Analysis of Recorded Cases of Phthisis Pulmonalis," *Transactions of the American Climatological Association,* Vol. VIII (1891), 73; Darlington, "The Doubtful Efficacy of a Hot, Dry Climate in Disease," *ibid.,* Vol. VIII (1891), 237; Wetherill, "Health-Resorts of the West and Southwest," *Medical News* (Philadelpia), Vol. LXIII (December 16, 1893), 681–83.

natives of the state, and issued a most revealing circular which concluded:

> A little while ago such a thing as the development of a case of consumption in Colorado was unknown. Now such instances are becoming more and more common. There is little doubt that these cases usually originate through careless association with consumptives. . . . People here must begin to protect themselves.[10]

And Dr. Milton J. Bleim, a staunch defender of Texas' climate, was forced in 1903 to admit that thousands of phthisics

> have been allowed, or encouraged to leave home, only to die among strangers, in loneliness and sorrow. The mortality records of San Antonio, Texas, show that 60 per cent of all deaths from tuberculosis occur within the first year of their residence there.[11]

By far the severest indictment of southwestern climates was recorded in 1906 by Albert Hale. "Twenty thousand new cases of consumption," he wrote, "come to the great Southwest every year . . . ."

> But a fearful proportion of these twenty thousand die here, away from home, strangers in a strange land, not always surrounded by even the simplest comforts, often in poverty, coughing their lives away, a burden to themselves, an expense to their friends, a care upon the charity of the community into which fate has thrown them.
>
> Twelve thousand of these twenty thousand consumptives die within the year. This is only a guess, but its accuracy cannot be denied, and if it errs, it is on the side of moderation.[12]

Why, Hale asked rhetorically, do 60 per cent of these newcomers perish? His succinct answer was—a continuing and ob-

[10] Colorado State Board of Health, *Circular No. 9: Consumption and How to Prevent Its Spread in Colorado*, 8.

[11] "The Influence of the Climate of Southwestern Texas Upon Respiratory Diseases," *North American Journal of Homeopathy*, Vol. LI (December, 1903), 746.

[12] "Tuberculosis: Climate and the Great Southwest," *The Reporter Magazine*, Vol. VII (1906), 135.

viously misplaced faith in the western health legend. He explained:

> . . . the vast majority of those who come . . . know nothing of the place, nothing of the essentials of a cure; they disregard or discard all requirements of treatment, and throw themselves helter-skelter, willy-nilly upon poor, long-suffering nature, recklessly deluding themselves into the belief that all will be well within a few . . . months, now that they have reached that panacea for every ill, a good climate.[13]

But, in all fairness, Hale noted that the fault rested not "with the legitimate promises which the great Southwest has made" but upon the "carelessness or cupidity of northern physicians, and upon the ignorance of many patients who might improve or recover if they went about it in the right way." Do not rely on climate alone, he pleaded; come while some hope of recovery still exists, and bring sufficient resources to provide for good food, adequate housing, and a prolonged rest. Only under these conditions could the climate of the Southwest be expected to act beneficially upon tuberculosis.

A great many men agreed with Hale that it was not the failure but the misuse of climate which had caused a sharp increase in mortality rates during the late nineteenth century. Most of them were convinced that a greater number of health-seekers improved when the Southwest was still a frontier because they were forced to co-operate more fully with the region's environmental elements. As early as 1872, John Tice wrote:

> Before railroads penetrated here [Colorado], when it took thirty to forty days to make the journey, more desperate cases were cured than now; because the strain on the lungs, caused by the increasing rarity of the air was so gradual that the slight lesions had time to heal.[14]

[13] *Ibid.*, 239.
[14] *Over the Plains and on the Mountains*, 153–54.

Dr. Charles Denison in 1876 used the same thesis in suggesting that consumptives approach the Rocky Mountains in stages. "A sojourn of a week," he wrote to those contemplating a winter's trip by rail,

> at some midway station (as at Wallace on the Kansas Pacific Railway), is advisable for some . . . invalids, or, better still, if in summer, a ride across the plains in a wagon, and camping out on the way.[15]

Similarly, Dr. Walter Jayne in 1888 begged phthisics to observe "two very simple rules": (1) approach elevated regions gradually and by easy stages, not in Pullman coaches; and (2) establish a continuous and prolonged residence. "I am confident," he concluded convincingly,

> were the first of these rules more generally followed, we should hear far less of the ill effects . . . and be able to note a larger percentage of advanced cases as improved; and if the second was faithfully observed, there would be more cures and fewer relapses.[16]

The need for a return to therapeutic, prairie-schooner traveling was still widely supported by doctors as late as 1895, but some tuberculars who put the advice into practice reaped extremely disappointing, even fatal, results.[17] The patient might willingly co-operate with western climates, but the obstinate bacillus too often would not.

Many eastern physicians also recommended (often to the consternation of those in the West who knew better) that patients

[15] "Report on the Climate of Colorado, and Its Relation to Pulmonary Diseases," *Transactions of the American Medical Association,* Vol. XXVII (1876), 462.

[16] "The Climate of Colorado and Its Effects," *Transactions of the American Climatological Association,* Vol. V (1888), 66.

[17] C. F. Nichols, M.D., "The Service of an Invalid Aid Society," *Review of Reviews* (New York), Vol. XI (March, 1895), 291; George L. Richards, M.D., *Consumption: Cases that Should Go to Colorado and Cases that Should Remain at Home,* 4–5.

"go West and rough it"; work on a ranch, they advised, or live in a tent in the great out-of-doors and meet nature on its own terms.[18] In many cases, such advice proved at least to be harmless if not always beneficial, for the accounts are legion of those who boasted of "wilderness cures." One of the more fortunate of this group even made a significant contribution to western culture; John B. Stetson, the consumptive son of a Philadelphia hatter, "roughed it" for two years in the Pikes Peak region and during that time fashioned the first of the now-famous Stetson hats, a high-domed, wide-brimmed headpiece which became a distinctive and traditional adjunct to the western man's riding habit.[19]

Increasingly the "ranch cure" technique became popular among pulmonary patients, but even so, western physicians like Samuel Fisk were quick to admonish the uninitiated that

> ranching life is necessarily somewhat rough . . . even a vigorous man . . . finds it most irksome and fatiguing. We think it a great mistake to increase the trials of an invalid by imposing on him . . . a life that is rough in the extreme, and a dietary innutritious, uninviting and monotonous. The average ranch-house is a miserable shanty, out on the plains, away from neighbors, where the usual diet is bacon floating in grease; hot flapjacks, made fresh with water and baking-powder, and coffee without milk.[20]

Doctors in the West were much more willing to admit the reliability of tent dwelling as a therapeutic practice, but only if it were dissociated from the notion of "roughing it." "While advising tent life," Dr. F. E. Waxham cautioned in 1902, "as a

[18] Henry Sewell, M.D., *Some Considerations on the Climatic Treatment of Consumption with Especial Reference to Denver as a Health Resort,* 4; Craig, "Open-Air Treatment of Tuberculosis: Tent Life in Arizona," *Journal of the American Medical Association,* Vol. XXXIX (October 4, 1902), 841.

[19] Tinkle and Maxwell, *The Cowboy Reader,* 121–22.

[20] "Colorado for Invalids," *Popular Science Monthly,* Vol. XXV (July, 1884), 318; Alfred Terry Bacon, "Ranch-Cure," *Lippincott's Magazine,* (n.s.) Vol. II (July, 1881), 90–96; F. H. Taylor, "Through Texas," *Harper's New Monthly Magazine,* Vol. LIX (October, 1879), 714.

means of obtaining the greatest amount of pure fresh air, yet we advise with it and as a part of the treatment, food, rest, and comfort."[21] He added emphatically that the strenuous activities of the healthy camper should form no part of an invalid's life and stated unequivocally that few physicians disputed the advisability of his recommendations.

Waxham spoke the truth, but the medical fraternity had reached this new plateau of harmony only after a painstaking decade of reappraising the whole concept of climatology. Slowly, however, even the most loosely kept statistics again proved the undeniable value of living in a situation where an abundance of fresh air was available night and day. Logically, tent life complemented the new consensus perfectly, and doctors responded to a growing demand for professionally approved canopies with several cleverly conceived designs.[22]

Thus tent therapy, almost by default, commanded greater attention by the turn of the century than any other technique in the treatment of tuberculosis, and in an interesting way, this trend represented for both physicians and patients another attempt to cling to the old climate-cure theory. Where once the deadly bacillus had threatened to brush aside all faith in a nature cure, the clinician's inability to produce a reliable specific for tuberculosis caused a retrenchment in medical opinion to a position similar to that of an earlier period. And the invalid, shunned in health centers and denied access to public and private housing, found in self-imposed tent isolation a new modicum of hope and a greater degree of acceptance in a health frontier grown restive by the presence of increasing numbers of consumptives.

As a general rule, the "triad treatment"—fresh air, nourishing

[21] "The Outdoor Treatment of Tuberculosis," *Journal of the American Medical Association,* Vol. XXXIX (November 29, 1902), 1393.

[22] See for example: Gardiner, "The Sanatory Tent and Its Use in the Treatment of Pulmonary Tuberculosis," *Transactions of the American Climatological Association,* Vol. XVIII (1902), 209–21; Denison, "The Sleeping Canopy," *ibid.,* Vol. XXIII (1907), 183–99.

food, and absolute rest—formed the basis of a medically approved tent regimen, but a not-too-surprising emphasis was again placed upon the necessity of selecting a location which permitted year-round exposure to a favorable climate. Some physicians recommended seasonal shifts, i.e., summers in Colorado and winters in New Mexico or Arizona, as the best means of assuring comfort as well as uninterrupted outdoor life. The greater number, however, expressed a definite preference for a continuous residence in the hot, dry regions of southwestern Texas, New Mexico, and Arizona.[23]

Tent cities designed exclusively for consumptives sprang up throughout the lower Southwest, and doctors gave hearty approval to their development since suitable companionship for the invalid was always present and some medical supervision of his habits was theoretically possible. Sunmount near Santa Fe, Tent City near Roswell, and Bugville near Tucson, were among the largest of these canvas-topped oases, but almost every town of any size in the Southwest had at least a modest community of tent dwellers.[24]

One of the most isolated of the smaller tent colonies was located near Fort Davis, Texas. Built just after the turn of the century by a pioneer resident, Will Pruett, the appropriately named "Tent City" consisted of a "frame recreation and dining hall, and 12 cottages with adobe walls and tenting roofs." Newspaper and pamphlet advertisements helped to make the resort a "going concern" by 1906, but inaccessibility doomed it to an early failure.

23 Waxham, "The Outdoor Treatment of Tuberculosis," *Journal of the American Medical Association,* Vol. XXXIX (November 19, 1902), 1393; Elliott, "A Practical View of Tent Life in the Southwest," *New York Medical Journal,* Vol. LXXXIV (October 6, 1906), 685–89; Edward E. Elliott, "Tenting for Health in the Desert: A Health-Seeker's Advice to Health-Seekers," *The World To-Day,* Vol. XII (April, 1907), 404–13.

24 Max Frost and Paul A. F. Walter (eds.), *The Land of Sunshine . . . (1904),* 111. Elliott, "A Practical View of Tent Life in the Southwest," *New York Medical Journal,* Vol. LXXXIV (October 6, 1906), 687; Rodgers, "Some Observations on Tuberculosis by a Dweller in the Desert," *Charities Review,* Vol. XVI (September 1, 1906), 562.

The camp's uniqueness was due to the use of an unusual therapeutic device known as an "inhalatorium," a glass and metal case which was large enough for an adult to stand in while breathing concentrated medicinal vapors. Now worn by time and obscured by history, only a few crumbled walls and personal reminiscences remain to give Pruett credit "for trying to aid sick humanity."[25]

The few conveniences and scant medical facilities available in tent camps seldom were inexpensive, and for that reason a great body of destitute consumptives always avoided them and ventured instead out onto the deserted plains and wastelands, the tent becoming as a result almost as commonplace in these regions as was the tipi half a century earlier. Traveling alone or in small groups, these nomadic "desert rats" were little more than prisoners of hope, constantly shifting their crude living quarters with changes in weather while clinging desperately to the last thread of life.[26] Farmers and ranchers were continually deluged with their requests for light employment or even for the privilege of camping near a homesite so that food and provisions might be easily obtained. But when all resources were exhausted or when death was imminent, these humble tuberculars converged on nearby cities and prostrated themselves before public and private charities for succor while they lived and for interment when they perished.

A serious social and economic burden fell upon the Southwest as demands for employment and charity rose in the early 1900's. Most healthy citizens so feared the invalid's presence that a concerted and easily recognizable resentment greeted the coming of each new wave of transient coughers. Ominous "Consumptives Not Accepted" signs, posted in hotels, boardinghouses, and restaurants, bore out clearly the extent of the expressed and un-

25 Barry Scobee, "History Obscures Tent City," San Angelo (Texas) *Standard-Times*, February 14, 1960.

26 Janet Brownell Glen, "Prisoners of Hope," *The Outlook*, Vol. LVII (October 23, 1897), 475.

compromising resistance offered by city merchants. Morale among workers in firms employing health-seekers was seriously undermined not only by the fear of infection but also by the fierce competition for jobs which frequently drove wage scales "below the living point." Gradually businessmen, as well as ranch and farm owners, felt obliged to refuse employment to tuberculars at any price, but in so doing they shifted an oppressive responsibility to public and private charities, whose limited funds became perennially exhausted.[27] Still, invalids came and the problem increased until, with uncommon but understandable bitterness, the Southwest revolted.

It was not difficult to single out for castigation the real villain in the Southwest's oppressive dilemma; certainly little or no blame could be attached to the poor, hopeless consumptive, for he was merely grasping for straws in a well-gleaned repertory of medical remedies for his distresses. Guilty instead, from either ignorance or malpractice, were the hundreds of eastern physicians who dispatched westward an unending stream of invalids who would inevitably die or become the wards of western communities.[28] Albert Hale was particularly severe in criticizing a group he referred to as "irredeemable" northern physicians:

> There are, of course, plenty of rascals in the profession. These rob their patients until they die, or until they escape, to drift forlornly into the Southwest, hoping that, impoverished as they are, they have not yet come too late. Then there are those who . . . get rid of their patients by ordering them away to die, out of sight, out of mind, or who sent their patients away so as to save their home statistics.[29]

[27] Sharlot M. Hall, "The Burden of the Southwest," *Out West,* Vol. XXVIII (January, 1908), 4–6; Hale, "Tuberculosis: Climate and the Great Southwest," *The Reporter Magazine,* Vol. VII (1906), 242.

[28] Warner W. Watkins, M.D., "Ignorance or Malpractice? Financial and Climatic Conditions in the Treatment of Tuberculosis," *Journal of the American Medical Association,* Vol. LII (April 10, 1909), 1175–76.

[29] "Tuberculosis: Climate and the Great Southwest," *The Reporter Magazine,* Vol. VII (1906), 240.

Similarly, Dr. Warner Watkins of Phoenix, Arizona, felt "that reputable physicians in every section of the country" were responsible for contributing to the increasing death ratio and the growing financial burdens of the Southwest. Half-dead and financially troubled consumptives, Watkins stated, ought to be kept at home in the most favorable surroundings. But he concluded despairingly:

> The custom is that, in the face of all known teachings concerning the disease and in the face of common sense and humanity, physicians will persist in sending this class of patient away from home, family, and friends to die in a strange land, by holding out to them the fatuous hope of recovery in a "change of climate." . . .
>
> Each winter the Associated Charities of . . . [Phoenix] is swamped with such a class of patients and the county hospital is filled with them, and our potter's field is a veritable monument to the guilt of all practitioners who are guilty of malpractice.[30]

The battle lines were drawn, and all the trappings of a full-fledged boycott of consumptives became clearly visible. If practitioners in the East insisted on making the Southwest a dumping ground for the nation's tuberculars, then suitable safeguards against such a practice had to be taken. Perhaps a turning point was reached in 1899 when an eastern physician, Dr. Leland Cofer, suggested "the formation of a colony of consumptives in California, to be recruited from the Eastern States, and supported by our wealthy, public-spirited citizens." Popular indignation in California rose promptly, and legislation was discussed which called for the quarantining of incoming consumptives, and even for the eventual exclusion of those who in the future might try to enter the state.[31] Such bluster went for naught, but other states thereafter joined California in varying responses to the problem thus identified.

[30] "Ignorance or Malpractice?" *Journal of the American Medical Association*, Vol. XII (April 10, 1909), 1176.

[31] Knopf, "The California Quarantine against Consumptives," *Forum*, Vol. XXVIII (January, 1900), 615–20.

Although no strong sentiment in favor of excluding consumptives arose in Colorado, invalids felt the sting of rejection in other ways. "The people of Colorado," Francis Kinder wrote in 1903,

> are not ungenerous in spirit, yet with a large class of consumptives among them, and the need of guarding against infection being so often emphasized by physicians and the press, a dread of the disease has grown so strong that the invalid can scarcely secure accommodations . . . . The matter of securing suitable employment . . . adds to the difficulties of the situation. With impaired physical strength, and with employers and employees prejudiced against his presence, the consumptive is indeed handicapped.[32]

In Texas, sentiment ran somewhat higher. The state's health officer, Dr. W. M. Brumby, issued the following official notice in 1909 to the nation's doctors:

> *Consumptives Unwelcome in Texas.* . . . the people of the state are no longer able to cope with the tuberculosis situation. So many consumptives have been sent to Texas that the death rate from that disease has risen from almost nothing to over 10 per cent., and that the natives are now suffering from the disease because the population is unable to assimilate the added consumptives. The local charitable associations are said to be impoverished and are unable to look after those now in Texas. . . . Almost all Texas hotels and private boarding houses refuse to accommodate consumptives.[33]

Only in New Mexico were tuberculars able to find prolonged encouragement. New Mexicans believed strongly in the ability of their climate to restore the ill and to protect the healthy, and the Territory's Bureau of Immigration continued for a time to make unreserved appeals to health-seekers. One announcement in 1906 read reassuringly:

[32] "The Consumptive's Chances in Colorado," *Review of Reviews* (New York), Vol. XXVII (June, 1903), 698.

[33] "Consumptives Unwelcome in Texas," *Journal of the American Medical Association,* Vol. LII (April 3, 1909), 1118.

> Health seekers are invited. New Mexico does not intend to shut the door upon them. . . . Ample accommodations are to be found at tent cities, hotels, sanitariums, and homes in the larger towns, as well as in the smaller settlements . . . and [the] various hot springs.[34]

Even the Land of Enchantment's enthusiasm was eventually dulled, however, by the same forces which had caused other southwestern states to rebel.

Unhappily, few, if any, of the restraining actions were very effective. State legislatures were hamstrung for constitutional reasons; they could do nothing to stop the flow of interstate travelers or even to quarantine transients without taking similar action against their own citizens. Nor did the dissuading tactics of hotel and residence owners appreciably reduce the annual volume of invalids. Most cities passed sanitary ordinances which required the disinfection of rooms occupied by tuberculars and prohibited indiscriminate spitting by infected persons, but even these ordinances went unobserved, largely because citizens refused to sanction the tax increases necessary to employ enough personnel for proper enforcement.[35]

By 1914, the entire Southwest admitted that it was incapable of dealing with a problem it then considered "interstate in proportion and properly one to be handled by federal authorities." Nine southwestern states in that year joined in requesting federal legislation "to provide hospitals for consumptives without means who come from other states seeking health." Governor Oscar B. Colquitt of Texas, at the request of the Southwestern Tuberculosis Conference, organized a ninety-nine-member committee composed of delegates appointed by the governors of Arizona,

[34] Frost and Walter, *The Land of Sunshine . . . (1906)*, 13.

[35] William P. Munn, "A Tuberculosis Quarantine Not Practical," *Forum*, Vol. XXIX (April, 1900), 185; Benedict, "Consumption Considered as a Contagious Disease," *Popular Science Monthly*, Vol. XLVIII (November, 1895), 37; Hale, "Tuberculosis: Climate and the Great Southwest," *The Reporter Magazine*, Vol. VII (1906), 243.

California, Colorado, Kansas, Nevada, New Mexico, Oklahoma, Texas, and Utah, a committee which gave vigorous support and sponsorship to the Shafroth-Calloway bill.[36]

Already under consideration by Congress, the bill provided that abandoned military reservations and other government property in the Southwest be reactivated as tuberculosis hospitals for indigent consumptives, and that the United States Public Health Service hospital at Fort Stanton, New Mexico, be used for any indigent consumptives who "have contracted their infection in another state and who by reasons of their affliction are a menace to interstate commerce."

Some of those who sympathized with the efforts of the Southwest felt the Shafroth-Calloway bill should be strengthened to provide that a "certain percentage of the cost of maintenance of an indigent lunger . . . be chargeable against his home town or county"; if this were done, they thought, officials and doctors would stop sending their patients away indiscriminately.[37] Unfortunately, many fancy words and all raised emotions were wasted; the Shafroth-Calloway bill, like much other progressive legislation, became engulfed by a bigger problem—world conflict—and it failed to pass.

The idea of creating sanatoria at old army forts in the Southwest was not without precedent. Such a notion was prominently associated with a movement in the early nineties calling for the establishment of a national sanatorium for indigent consumptives. In response to increasing public interest in this regard, a bill, first introduced in 1891 by Representative William Cogswell of Massachusetts and later under joint authorship with Senator Jacob Gallinger of New Hampshire, actually placed such a proposal before Congress. The Joint Resolution called for a team of physicians, appointed by the President, to survey abandoned gov-

36 "The Problem of Poor Lungers Who Go West," *The Survey*, Vol. XXXII (April 18, 1914), 67.

37 *Ibid.*

ernment reservations in western territories with a view toward creation of a federally financed sanatorium. In addition, the American Invalid Society of New England a few years later requested permission to establish a consumptive hospital at Fort Marcy, New Mexico.[38]

These and other pieces of legislation relating to public health succumbed, like Shafroth-Calloway in a later period, to war fever; "when the war with Spain was declared," U. O. B. Wingate observed in 1898, "an end to all such legislation resulted."[39] Much of the enthusiasm for a national sanatorium waned in the years that followed, but Congress in 1899 did authorize the establishment of service-controlled tubercular hospitals at Forts Bayard and Stanton in New Mexico.

Fort Stanton, several miles distant from Roswell, was used by the United States Public Health and Marine Hospital Service (Department of the Treasury) as a sanatorium for "seamen employed on vessels of the merchant marine of the United States, keepers and crews of lighthouses, officers and men of the Revenue Cutter Service and the Coast and Geodetic Survey, and officers and men employed on government vessels other than navy." Dr. Paul M. Carrington, a consumptive in the first stage when he arrived at the fort, assumed command of the renovated facilities and recovered from the disease after a residence of only two years. He formulated a therapeutic program, based on the triad treatment, which helped countless seamen win back their health.[40]

Fort Bayard near Silver City was reactivated as the United

[38] William Thornton Parker, "Shall We Have a National Sanitarium for Consumptives?" *The Arena,* Vol. XVI (July, 1896), 202–203; Keleher, *Turmoil in New Mexico 1846–1868,* 119.

[39] U. O. B. Wingate, "National Health Legislation," *North American Review,* Vol. CXLVII (November, 1898), 529.

[40] Oliver P. Newman, "Government Care of Consumptives," *Review of Reviews* (New York), Vol. XXX (July, 1904), 59–61; Carrington, "The Climate of New Mexico—Nature's Sanatorium for Consumptives," *Transactions of the American Climatological Association,* Vol. XXIII (1907), 83–88; Frank D. Reeve, *History of New Mexico,* II, 283.

States General Hospital for the treatment of "officers and men of the army and navy who have contracted tuberculosis in the government service." Major D. M. Appel, an army surgeon with an advanced case of phthisis, became the first director of the hospital and employed with equal success the triad formula in restoring scores of diseased military personnel to active service. Appel himself recovered so satisfactorily that after six years of service at Bayard, he was reassigned to regular duty and was stationed in the Philippines.[41]

These forts, once noble vanguards turned ignoble servants of the frontier, were carefully controlled by their respective service organizations during their early existence and therefore were not open to the general public. Consequently, their influence was confined to areas other than that of relieving the physical pressure then being exerted upon western health facilities. In addition to providing much-needed medical care for merchant marine and military servicemen, both hospitals pioneered a special tent-house development which was copied extensively throughout the Southwest. Both also, with typical bureaucratic efficiency, kept copious records and statistics which ultimately became valuable mirrors of a successfully applied therapeutic program. Moreover, experience at Stanton and Bayard proved the unquestioned value of regimented supervision in treating tuberculosis.[42]

A gratifying increase in private sanatoria, financed by religious, fraternal, and charitable organizations, appeared in the Southwest after the turn of the century. Most of them were operated exclusively by and for a particular group, but they nonetheless struck at the very core of a beleaguered region's major problem. Collections of such hospitals were to be found at Phoe-

[41] Newman, "Government Care of Consumptives," *Review of Reviews* (New York, Vol. XXX (July, 1904), 64; Appel, "The Army Hospital and Sanitorium for the Treatment of Tuberculosis, at Fort Bayard, New Mexico," *Journal of the American Medical Association,* Vol. XXXIX (November 29, 1902), 1373–79.

[42] E. S. Bullock, M.D., and C. T. Sands, M.D., "Twelve Years of Pulmonary Tuberculosis Treatment in the West," *ibid.,* Vol. LII (June 19, 1909), 1974–75.

nix and Tucson in Arizona, at Albuquerque in New Mexico, at El Paso and San Antonio in Texas, and at Denver and Colorado Springs in Colorado. And these health centers, too numerous to mention individually, were founded by such church groups as Baptist, Catholic, Dutch Reformed, Jewish, Lutheran, and Methodist; such fraternal or professional orders as Modern Woodmen of America, Swedish Nationals, International Typographical Union, and International Stereotypers and Electrotypers Union of North America; and such civil affiliates as the Junior League and organized charities.[43]

Accompanying the development of private hospitals was an expansion of county and municipal health facilities, most of which provided improvised isolation wards for at least a few tubercular patients. By 1912 one southwestern state, Texas, created a state tuberculosis sanatorium at Carlsbad in Tom Green County, an establishment which operates at present under the name of McKnight State Sanatorium. In addition, the United States Indian Service, after 1910, constructed half a dozen consumptive aid stations on widely scattered Indian reservations in Arizona, Nevada, and New Mexico.[44] Collectively the number of these new developments seems imposing, but their combined capacity perennially fell far short of total demand.

An eastern-inspired "sanatorium-movement" brought gradual but increasing relief. This was partially a response to the Southwest's persistent pleas of "keep the indigent consumptive at home," partly a product of an increased feeling of civic responsibility toward resident phthisics, but in greater part the result of surmise that all fresh air possesses the same revivifying qualities;[45]

[43] National Tuberculosis Association, *A Directory of Sanatoria, Hospitals, Day Camps, and Preventoria for the Treatment of Tuberculosis in the United States,* 2–4, 18–22, 76–78, 122–26.

[44] W. P. Webb, *Handbook of Texas,* II, 118–19; National Tuberculosis Association, *A Directory of Sanatoria,* 2–4, 70–71, 77–78.

[45] Adams, "Tuberculosis: The Real Race Suicide," *McClure's Magazine,* Vol. XXIV (January, 1905), 249; Henry I Bowditch, "Open-Air Travel as a Curer

the movement gained momentum through the years until the East's diversified accommodations for tuberculars—cottages, day camps, sanatoria, preventoria, and hospitals—exceeded in capacity those in the West.

The acknowledged pioneer of the sanatorium movement was Dr. Edward L. Trudeau of New York. This medical humanitarian, who spent most of his life trying to check the spread of tuberculosis, opened in 1883 the semi-charitable Adirondack Cottage Sanatorium near Saranac Lake, an institution built philanthropically by New York donors, staffed gratuitously by some of the state's most prominent physicians, and superintended voluntarily by "gentlemen residing in the Adirondack region for health." Constructed according to the "cottage plan"—several two- to four-patient cottages clustered around a commodious mess, recreation, and isolation ward building—the institution catered to consumptives of moderate means, the major expense being defrayed by yearly subscriptions from "benevolent persons" and the balance by nominal weekly payments from the patients.[46]

The sanatorium's success was instantaneous, its reputation nationwide, but its duplication all too slow. By 1905, only 135 institutions of all types could be counted in "thirty-three states and provinces of the United States and Canada where tuberculosis patients [were] cared for," but interested physicians were encouraged by the fact that fifty-four of these establishments had been constructed between 1902 and 1904. Significantly, one-third of all such structures by that time were located in New York and Pennsylvania.[47]

and Preventer of Consumption, as Seen in the History of a New England Family," *Science*, Vol. XIV (October 4, 1889), 230–32.

[46] Alfred L. Loomis, M.D., "Presidential Address," *Transactions of the American Climatological Association*, Vol. II, (1885), 3–4. Loomis was an examining and consulting physician for the sanitarium.

[47] Livingston Farrand, "The First Annual Meeting of the National Association for the Study and Prevention of Tuberculosis, Washington, D.C., May 18 and 19, 1905," *Charities Review*, Vol. XIV (June 3, 1905), 803.

A new face was added in the early 1900's when tents were incorporated into the sanatorium movement. By adding a large number of tent cottages to the Metropolitan Hospital's permanent installations, the New York commissioner of public charities, in conjunction with the hospital, in 1902 opened what became the largest facility for consumptives in New York City.[48] In 1903, two isolated tent colonies were opened at Liberty, New York, under the general supervision of Dr. Edward Stubbert, himself a restored tubercular. One of these camps, the Piney Woods Inn, was an extension of a boardinghouse, the owner of which rented individual tents for outdoor living and provided nourishing meals in the inn at a total cost of not more than ten dollars a week. The other camp, completely improvised, consisted of tents of varying sizes arranged around a master canopy, which served in the same capacity as the inn.[49] Officials throughout the East soon learned that tents provided the most economical accommodation for money-conscious invalids.

Extensive use thereafter was made of canvas structures to provide temporary and much needed shelter for people of meager means. The Boston Association for the Relief and Control of Tuberculosis, borrowing upon an idea first implemented in Berlin, Germany, developed in 1905 "an open air day camp for consumptives," an unusual tent-dwelling arrangement operated exclusively for Boston's destitute classes. Patients came from all parts of the city to spend eight hours daily in a tightly organized program of hygiene consisting of appropriate foods, adequate rest, and meaningful recreation—all at a cost of only forty cents a day exclusive of transportation. In addition, lectures were given at intervals by leading physicians on how the afflicted might avoid communicating the disease to other members of their families.[50]

48 "Tent Cottages for Consumptives," *ibid.*, Vol. X (May 9, 1903), 518.

49 J. Edward Stubbert, M.D., "Tent Life for Consumptives," *Transactions of the American Climatological Association*, Vol. XIX (1903), 93–94.

50 "The Boston Day Camp for Consumptives," *Charities Review*, Vol. XIV

The day camp development became a widely copied plan throughout the major eastern cities.

The total effect of the sanatorium movement was immense. By the outbreak of World War I, sufficient facilities were available to encourage a large proportion of eastern consumptives to remain at home, and enough success had been enjoyed in treating them in home climates to make physicians want to keep them there. The greatest effects were felt within the poorer classes; they were no longer willing to leave municipal conveniences, families, and friends to journey westward to face wilderness deprivation, resistance, and frequently death among strangers. The well to do bridged inconvenience and rejection with affluence and prestige; for them the door was never closed.

It took some time for the momentum of three-quarters of a century to abate, and the Southwest continued for at least two decades to accommodate diminishing numbers of transient coughers. But by then the legend of perfect health in the West was gone, largely because the premise on which it was based had been destroyed by a deadly micro-organism, one which seemed oblivious to all legends, climates, and even medicines.

Thus the West's greatest bonanza was finally playing out, but it is significant to note that the sharpest "line of demarcation" in the change from climate cures to home treatments was, as Samuel Fisk noted, "the pocket-book."[51] As soon as (but not until) adequate low-cost therapy was available in the East, westward migrations declined. Throughout this transition, however, the West's claim to the more rejuvenating climate suffered very little; enlightened physicians everywhere continued to acknowledge the superiority of the climates of Arizona, New Mexico, South-

(July 29, 1905), 961; Alexander M. Wilson, "A Summer Camp for Tuberculosis," *ibid.*, 1045.

[51] See the discussions following Bonney, "Discussions Upon 'Climatic Treatment of Pulmonary Tuberculosis *versus* Home Sanatoria'," *Transactions of the American Climatological Association*, Vol. XVII (1901), 228.

west Texas, Colorado, and southern California in treating respiratory diseases. As one eastern practitioner put in succinctly: "If we the physicians were the patients" and it came to a question of "whether we would go to the best climate when we had tuberculosis, we would every one answer yes."[52]

[52] See for example Stubbert, "Tent Life for Consumptives," *ibid.*, Vol. XIX (1903), 95; and the discussions following Bonney, "Discussions upon 'Climatic Treatment of Pulmonary Tuberculosis versus Home Sanatoria,' " *ibid.*, Vol. XVII (1901), 234.

IX. *And Still They Come*

THE HEYDAY of the health frontier and of climatotherapy was over by 1900. More and more the bug of contagion crawled into the pattern of medical thought; less and less did physicians ponder the question of which climate answers best. "The age of the tourist lasted," one author wrote reflectively about the period 1891–1918, "but the medical profession began to change the prescription for the treatment of tuberculosis by putting their patients to bed at home instead of sending them . . . 'to eat and sleep in the out of doors.' "[1]

What remains of the age of invalidism is still easily discernible but is nonetheless largely forgotten. Why forgotten? Perhaps the odium of fear and resentment which surrounded the dreaded tubercular was so strong that many southwesterners, with Freudian ease, have attempted unconsciously to make others forget the climatic benefits which come to residents in the region. Perhaps the later health-seekers deliberately and deceitfully withheld the truth of their condition in order to escape discrimination and rejection. Or perhaps the sparkling successes of modern medicines have so completely reoriented medical theories and practices that the old climate-cure notion has been almost wholly disregarded.

[1] Carter, *The Pikes Peak Region,* 30.

Probabilities, however, fall short of telling the complete story. Of greater significance is the fact that after 1900 the search for health ceased to be a major factor in the development of the Southwest; the region's economy became so diversified that dwindling invalid dollars were scarcely missed and not particularly needed. For resort promoters and merchants it was simply a case of "out of sight, out of mind."

For the most part, even the folklore of western invalidism disappeared. Memory-perpetuating legends, so important in shaping the traditions of trapping, trading, mining, and ranching, failed to survive the passing of the health-seeker's frontier, and twentieth century Americans, propelled by world events from one major crisis to another, find it increasingly difficult, without such tales, to recall the consumptive's glamourless, unexciting search for personal health.

Telltale signs of that age still exist nonetheless. Simple place designations such as Mentone in California and Carlsbad in New Mexico, both named in the nineteenth century after popular European resort centers, are typical, if ignored, reminders of the period. Malaria, still a problem disease in low-lying, semitropical regions of the world, is the most meaningful residue of a misguided era of miasmatic medicine; the word malaria itself means "bad air." And how minimize the persistent and lingering faith in the use of medicinal and thermal waters everywhere? Or how overlook the steady stream of asthmatics who annually find incontestable relief in the arid sections of the greater Southwest?

It is unfortunate that time, the greatest obscurer, has dealt so harshly with the health-seekers; for their contributions were, and continue to be, truly significant. From the standpoint of population alone, the search for health was a factor second only to the desire for land in attracting permanent settlers to the Southwest; easily 20 per cent of those who emigrated to the region between 1870 and 1900 were hopeful invalids, and that figure does not include perhaps an even larger number of transients who sought relief in the region's commercialized watering places.[2]

Southwestern states (as well as the entire nation) profited greatly from their coming. A. A. Hayes, Jr., noted in 1881 that former invalids were "an element in society entirely different from the pioneers, but they are very useful and important citizens . . . and are making their presence and influence strongly felt." And Sharlot Hall observed in 1908 that "the most useful citizens in many a community came there for health, and, having found it, chose to cast their lot with the land. Wealth, energy, culture, and trained ability came with the health seeker."[3]

Health-seekers were indeed a true cross section of American life, and their contributions were as varied as the colors of a prism. Most of them became "westerners" only because they traveled in a westerly direction during their quests for health; always their social and cultural tastes were dictated by those cultivated previously in eastern settings. Some of them were well-educated individuals and highly successful businessmen who, after their arrival, promptly filled the professional ranks,[4] built charitable health centers,[5] developed fashionable vacation cen-

[2] According to census figures, between 1870 and 1900 the total population of seven southwestern states and territories increased by 3,821,482 people, mostly through immigration. Included in that number were approximately three-quarters of a million health-seekers. For a quick reference on cumulative census reports, see E. Eastman Irvine (ed.), *The World Almanac and the Book of Facts for 1945,* 460.

[3] "Pioneers of the Sierra Madre," *International Review,* Vol. X (June, 1881), 523; Hall, "The Burden of the Southwest," *Out West,* Vol. XXVIII (January, 1908), 6.

[4] See for example Gardiner, *Doctor at Timberline,* 8–10.

[5] Frank M. Craig, "scion of an illustrious Pennsylvania family dating from Colonial days," coughed his way to Denver in 1907, encountered other "derelict" tuberculars who needed help, and founded shortly thereafter the Brotherly Relief Colony (later Craig Colony) at nearby Edgewater. See Meredith Davis, "Love, Faith and Life: the Story of the Invalid Who Was the Founder of Denver's Craig Colony," *Sunset,* Vol. XLIV (April, 1920), 62–64.

ters,[6] and provided political and civic leadership at all levels of government.

A few restored invalids rose even to national political prominence in the twentieth century. For example, New York–born, Harvard-educated Bronson Murray Cutting was brought to New Mexico "on a stretcher" in 1910 and "literally rose from the grave" to become a powerful and influential United States Senator (1929–35). Unfortunately a fatal airplane accident in Missouri on May 6, 1935, brought a tragic end to a life which tuberculosis could not conquer. Tuberculosis also drove Clinton Presba Anderson from South Dakota to New Mexico in 1917, but Anderson lost little time in making his presence known. After successes in business and civic organizations, he was elected to Congress in 1940, was appointed secretary of agriculture in 1945 by President Harry Truman, and was elevated to the Senate in 1949. He currently heads the all-important Senate Aeronautical and Space Sciences Committee. And previously mentioned John Nance Garner of Texas rose from a small town (Uvalde) legal practice to the vice-presidency of the United States (1933–41).[7]

Finally, two of the most prominent contemporary southwesterners are the sons of former invalids. Carl Trumbell Hayden, whose New England father (Charles T. Hayden) first recovered

[6] F. O. Stanley, an eastern engineer, architect, man of letters, and co-inventor of the famous Stanley Steamer, was sent to Colorado in 1903 by doctors who hoped to prolong his life for "a year or so." He survived for thirty-seven years and died at the age of ninety-three. Becoming impressed with the soothing climate of Estes Park, he helped other residents of the park to develop its resort aspects. When Stanley could not persuade the railroads to build a trunk line into the area, he then constructed a highway at his own expense and operated a fleet of Stanley Steamers from Lyons (the closest rail head) into Estes Park. Edwin J. Foscue and Louis O. Quam, *Estes Park: Resort in the Rockies,* 52–54.

[7] *Memorial Services Held in the House of Representatives . . . in Eulogy of Bronson Cutting, Late Senator From New Mexico,* 45; "On Sen. Clinton P. Anderson: Anderson to Succeed Kerr as Space Committee Chairman," *Congressional Quarterly Fact Sheet,* January 21, 1963, p. 1. Another health-seeker, Theodore Roosevelt, achieved even greater political heights, but his quest for health took him no farther south than North Dakota. See Baur, "The Health Seeker in the Westward Movement," 108.

from "lung-fever" at Old Point Comfort, Virginia, and later made his residence at Tuscon, Arizona, is currently the oldest ranking member and president pro tempore of the United States Senate. And Barry Morris Goldwater, former senator from Arizona and Republican candidate for President of the United States in 1964, is the son of Josephine Williams Goldwater, a consumptive but indomitable pioneer lady who actually hitchhiked her way to healthful Phoenix at the turn of the century.[8]

Prominent in their own fields but perhaps less spectacular in their achievements are several other twentieth-century sanatorians. Authors such as Harold Bell Wright, Ross Calvin, Kyle Crichton, and Edith Nicholl Ellison; journalists such as George Fitzpatrick, Ernie Pyle, J. Wesley Huff, Frances Rosser Brown, and James Swinnerton; businessmen such as Grover Hubbell, a member of an important financial family in Des Moines, Iowa, and Samuel Bixby, the "shoe polish king of his day"; and Dr. Howard Raper, "the inventor of X-ray film for mouth motion pictures of the teeth,"—all sought renewed health through periodic visits or by permanent residence in the Southwest.[9] And each of these men repaid his debt to Nature's natural sanatorium with gifts from his God-given talents.

None has done so more appropriately, however, than a lowly but spritely Roman Catholic priest—one Father Stanley, nee Stanley Francis Louis Crocchiola, presently ministering at Pep, Texas. In addition to being one of the most prolific researchers and chroniclers of New Mexican history, Father Stanley also tells

[8] Senator Carl Hayden to Jones, April 1, 1963, Jones Correspondence Files; Richard B. Stolley, "The Senator's [Barry Goldwater's] Pioneer Mother Talks About Barry and Herself," *Life,* Vol. LV (July 12, 1963), 25–26.

[9] George Fitzpatrick (ed.), *This is New Mexico,* 105, 126, 201, 236, 273, 286; Edith M. Nicholl, *Observations of a Ranchwoman in New Mexico,* 1–19; Edith Nicholl Ellison, *The Desert and the Rose,* foreword, 174ff; Senator Clinton P. Anderson to Jones, April 10, 1963, Jones Correspondence Files. Adam Clark Vroman, a prominent southwestern landscape photographer, developed a keen interest in the region after he brought his tubercular wife to Pasadena at the turn of the century. Ruth I. Mahood, *Photographer of the Southwest,* 12.

a very convincing and highly interesting story of the healthful attributes of southwestern climes:

> . . . I was teaching in St. John's College about 25 years ago when doctors found 2 spots on my right lung. They gave me 5 years if I didn't go to a dryer climate. This is how I first went to New Mexico—later Texas—I am still around and have had no recurrence of the condition. I have heard of others with the same experience. I also know of others that thought they were cured and returned only to die. Had they remained either in Texas, New Mexico, or Arizona they might have had more time. Fr. Gutierrez —who became pastor in Amarillo, Raton, Taos Hospital (Chaplain) was ordained so that he could say one Mass before he died. He came to New Mexico and Texas—has survived 57 years. I understand he is quite ill now and ready to die. He is 83 years old. Fr. Miller of Tome also came to this area after World War I with a lung condition. He is still active and happy in his work and looks quite healthy.[10]

The number of Stanley's published books and pamphlets already has reached a phenomenal level—an humble ecclesiastic's restitution to the Southwest for so great a physical blessing, his renewed health.

Thus the search for health plays a continuing, if diminishing, role in the development of the Southwest, and though a great part of the region's climatic attractiveness remains untarnished, most of the memories of the golden age of invalidism have long since dissipated. Throughout its prolonged history, the health frontier has served as a refuge for hundreds of thousands of uprooted invalids, and has in turn reaped many rewards from this grateful, talented, and resourceful group who traveled in search of life's greatest treasure—health.

[10] To Jones, May 14, 1963, Jones Correspondence Files.

Bibliography

ALL SOURCES used for this manuscript are published materials with the exception of a small amount of correspondence which the author had with certain contemporary health-seekers. These letters, in each case, are cited as being in the Jones Correspondence Files and are in the possession of the author. Also with rare exception, sources are primary in nature, a fact which makes impractical the bibliographical divisions normally contained in the reference section of a work of this type. In order to render the literature of the health-seeker as usable as possible, a simple arrangement has been employed—an alphabetical listing by author or, if anonymous, by title—and the entries are consistent with those used in the footnotes.

Abbott, George E., M.D. "Southern California Foot Hills," *Transactions of the American Climatological Association,* Vol. XVIII (1902), 96–102.

Abert, J. W. *Report . . . of His Examination of New Mexico, in the Years 1846–47,* 30 Cong., 1 sess., *Sen. Exec. Doc. 23.*

Adams, Samuel Hopkins. "Tuberculosis: The Real Race Suicide," *McClure's Magazine,* Vol. XXIV (January, 1905), 234–49.

Alden, C. H., M.D. "Some Southern California Health Resorts,"

Transactions of the American Climatological Association, Vol. XXI (1905), 44–54.

Allen, Paul, ed. *History of the Expedition under the Command of Captains Lewis and Clark to the Sources of the Missouri, Thence Across the Rocky Mountains and Down the River Columbia to the Pacific Ocean.* Philadelphia and New York, Bradford and Inskeep, 1814.

American Medical Association. *National Congress on Medical Quackery, October, 6–7, 1961.* Chicago, 1961.

Anderson, B. P., M.D. "Colorado as a Health Resort," *New York Medical Record,* Vol. XXXIII (March 17, 1888), 314–15.

Anderson, C. L. G., M.D. "Arizona as a Health Resort," *New York Medical Record,* Vol. XXXVIII (July 5, 1890), 8–10.

Appel, D. M., M.D. "The Army Hospital and Sanitorium for the Treatment of Tuberculosis, at Fort Bayard, New Mexico," *Journal of the American Medical Association,* Vol. XXXIX (November 29, 1902), 1373–79.

Ashe, Thomas. "Travels in America Performed in 1806, etc." In Lindley's *Indiana as Seen by Early Travelers, q.v.*

Atchison, Topeka and Santa Fe Railway Co. *Las Vegas Hot Springs, New Mexico.* Chicago, 1887.

Atkinson, Donald T. *Magic, Myth, and Medicine.* Cleveland and New York, The World Publishing Co., 1956.

Austin, Stephen F. *The Austin Papers.* Ed. by Eugene C. Barker. Vols. I and II, *Annual Report* of the American Historical Association for the Years 1919 and 1922, Washington, 1924, 1928; Vol. III, Austin, University of Texas Press, 1926.

———. "Descriptions of Texas, 1828," *Southwestern Historical Quarterly,* Vol. XXVIII (October, 1924), 104–20.

Ayer, I. Winslow. *Life in the Wilds of America, and Wonders of the West in and Beyond the Bounds of Civilization.* Grand Rapids, Mich., privately printed, 1880.

Bacon, Alfred Terry. "Ranch-Cure," *Lippincott's Magazine,* [n.s.] Vol. II (July, 1881), 90–96.

Baker, Henry B., M.D. "Relations of Certain Meteorological Conditions to Diseases of the Lungs and Air-Passages in Colorado," *Transactions of the American Climatological Association,* Vol. VII (1890), 210–38.

Bancroft, Frederick J., M.D. "About Health Resorts," *Magazine of Western History* (New York), Vol. XI (December, 1889), 171–73.

Bancroft, Hubert Howe. *History of Nevada, Colorado, and Wyoming 1540–1888.* Vol. XXV of *The Works of Hubert Howe Bancroft.* 39 vols. San Francisco, The History Co. 1886–90.

Bandelier, Adolf Francis Alphonse. "Why New Mexico Does Not Flourish," *The Nation,* Vol. XLII (January 28, 1886), 70–71.

Baur, John E. "The Health Seeker in the Westward Movement, 1830–1900," *Mississippi Valley Historical Review,* Vol. XLVI (June, 1959), 91–110.

———. *The Health Seekers of Southern California 1870–1900.* San Marino, Calif., The Huntington Library, 1959.

Beadle, J. H. *The Undeveloped West: or, Five Years in the Territories.* Philadelphia, Chicago, Cincinnati, St. Louis; National Publishing Co., 1873.

———. *Western Wilds and the Men Who Redeem Them.* Cincinnati, Jones Brothers and Co., 1877.

Beale, Edward F. *Wagon Road from Fort Defiance to the Colorado River,* 35 Cong., 1 sess., *House Exec. Doc. 124.*

Bell, William A. *New Tracks in North America: A Journal of Travel and Adventure Whilst Engaged in the Survey for a Southern Railroad to the Pacific Ocean During 1867–8.* 2 vols. London, Chapman and Hall, 1869.

Beltrami, Giacomo Constantino. *A Pilgrimage in Europe and America Leading to the Discovery of the Sources of the Mis-*

sissippi and Bloody Rivers; with a Description of the Whole Course of the Former and the Ohio. London, Hunt and Clarke, 1828.

Benedict, A. L., M.D. "Consumption Considered as a Contagious Disease," *Popular Science Monthly,* Vol. XLVIII (November, 1895), 33–39.

Berkeley, Grantley F. *The English Sportsman in the Western Prairies.* London, Hurst and Blackett, 1861.

Bett, Walter R. and others. *The History and Conquest of Common Diseases.* Norman, University of Oklahoma Press, 1954.

Bickham, William D. *From Ohio to the Rocky Mountains.* Dayton, Journal Book and Job Printing House, 1879.

Bidwell, John. *Echoes of the Past about California.* Ed. by Milo Milton Quaife. Chicago, R. R. Donnelley and Sons Co., 1928.

———. [Journal of a Trip to California in 1841]. [Weston, Mo., 1844?]

Bieber, Ralph Paul, ed. *The Southwest Historical Series.* 12 vols. Glendale, The Arthur H. Clark Co., 1931–43.

Bird, Isabella L. *A Lady's Life in the Rocky Mountains.* London, John Murray, 1879.

Birkbeck, Morris. "Notes on a Journey . . . to the Territory of Illinois (1818)." In Lindley's *Indiana as Seen by Early Travelers, q.v.*

Blaney, William Newnham. "An Excursion Through the U.S. and Canada 1822–23." As abridged in Lindley's *Indiana as Seen by Early Travelers, q.v.*

Bleim, Milton J., M.D. "The Influence of the Climate of Southwestern Texas Upon Respiratory Diseases," *North American Journal of Homeopathy,* Vol. LI (December, 1903), 746–51.

———. "The Place of Southwest Texas in Climate Therapeutics," *Medical Century* (Chicago), Vol. II (November 15, 1894), 521–26.

Bollaert, William. *William Bollaert's Texas.* Ed. by Eugene W.

Hollon and Ruth Lapham Butler. Norman, University of Oklahoma Press, 1956.

Bonney, Sherman G., M.D. "Discussion upon 'Climatic Treatment of Pulmonary Tuberculosis versus Home Sanatoria,'" *Transactions of the American Climatological Association,* Vol. XVII (1901), 224–34.

———. "When Should the Consumptive Residing in Colorado be Permitted to Return Home?" *Transactions of the American Climatological Association,* Vol. XVIII (1902), 203–207.

Bosley, Mary S., ed. *Hand-Book of Useful Knowledge: Comprising a Valuable Selection of Recipes in Medicine, Choice Things in Cookery, New Ideas in Gardening, etc., etc.* Philadelphia, Samuel B. Collins, 1881.

"The Boston Day Camp for Consumptives," *Charities Review,* Vol. XIV (July 29, 1905), 961.

Bowditch, Henry I., M.D. "Open-Air Travel as a Curer and Preventer of Consumption, as Seen in the History of a New England Family," *Science,* Vol. XIV (October 4, 1889), 230–32.

Bowditch, Vincent Y., M.D. "Home Treatment *versus* Climatic Treatment of Phthisis," *Transactions of the American Climatological Association,* Vol. XVII (1901), 214–18.

Bowles, Samuel. *Across the Continent.* Springfield, Mass., Samuel Bowles and Co., 1865.

———. *The Switzerland of America: A Summer Vacation in the Parks and Mountains of Colorado.* Springfield, Mass., Samuel Bowles and Co., 1869.

Bracht, Viktor. *Texas in 1848.* Trans. by Charles Frank Schmidt. San Antonio, The Naylor Printing Co., 1931.

Bradbury, John. *Travels in the Interior of America in the Years 1809, 1810, and 1811; including a Description of Upper Louisiana, Together with the States of Ohio, Kentucky, Indiana and Tennessee, with Illinois and Western Territories.* Liverpool, privately printed, 1817.

Brewerton, G. Douglas, "Incidents of Travel in New Mexico," *Harper's New Monthly Magazine,* Vol. VIII (April, 1854), 577–96.

Bridenbaugh, Carl. "Baths and Watering Places of Colonial America," *The William and Mary Quarterly* [3d series], Vol. III (April, 1946), 151–81.

Bridge, Norman, M.D. "The Climate of Southern California," *Transactions of the American Climatological Association,* Vol. XVII (1901), 85–96.

Brockett, L. P. *Our Western Empire: New West Beyond the Mississippi.* Philadelphia, Bradley, Garretson and Co., 1881.

Brown, Samuel R. "The Western Gazetteer; or Emigrant's Directory." In Lindley's *Indiana as Seen by Early Travelers, q.v.*

Browne, J. Ross. *Adventures in the Apache Country: A Tour Through Arizona and Sonora with Notes on the Silver Regions in Nevada.* New York, Harper and Brothers, 1869.

———. "A Tour Through Arizona," *Harper's New Monthly Magazine,* Vol. XXIX (October, 1864), 553–74.

Buley, R. Carlyle. *The Old Northwest: Pioneer Period: 1815–1840.* 2 vols. Bloomington, Ind., Indiana University Press, 1951.

Bulkley, L. Duncan, M.D. "Climate as It Affects the Skin and Its Diseases," *Transactions of the American Climatological Association,* Vol. XV (1899), 108–17.

Bullock, E. S., M.D., "The Southwest as a Resort for Pulmonary Patients," *Journal of the Outdoor Life* (National Tuberculosis Association), Vol. III (Saranac Lake, N.Y., 1906–1907), 46–48.

——— and C. T. Sands, M.D. "Twelve Years of Pulmonary Tuberculosis Treatment in the West," *Journal of the American Medical Association,* Vol. LII (June 19, 1909), 1973–80.

Bullock, W. *Sketch of a Journey Through the Western States of North America.* Vol. XIX of Thwaites' *Early Western Travels, q.v.*

Burke, Richard M. *An Historical Chronology of Tuberculosis.* 2d ed., Springfield, Ill., Charles C. Thomas, 1955.

Burnet, David G. "David G. Burnet's Letters Describing the Comanche Indians," with an Introduction by Ernest Wallace, West Texas Historical Association *Year Book,* Vol. XXX (October, 1954), 115–40.

Burns, William G., M.D. "Climate of Arizona," *Transactions of the American Climatological Association,* Vol. XVIII (1902), 241–46.

Burt, S. W., and E. L. Berthoud. *The Rocky Mountain Gold Regions.* Denver City, Jefferson Territory, Rocky Mountain News Printing Co., 1861.

Buttrick, Tilly, Jr. *Voyages, Travels and Discoveries, etc.* Vol. VIII of Thwaites' *Early Western Travels, q.v.*

C. W. Post: A Memorial. [Battle Creek, Mich., 1914?].

Carpenter, Frank D. Y. "The Climate Cure," *Lippincott's Magazine,* Vol. XXXI (April, 1883), 394–401.

Carrington, Paul M., M.D. "The Climate of New Mexico—Nature's Sanatorium for Consumptives," *Transactions of the American Climatological Association,* Vol. XXIII (1907), 71–100.

———. "Economic Housing of Consumptives, with Special Reference to the Southwest," *New York Medical Journal,* Vol. LXI (April 10, 1909), 421–30.

Carson, Thomas. *Ranching, Sport and Travel.* London and Leipsic, T. Fisher Unwin, 1911.

Carter, Harvey L., ed. *The Pikes Peak Region: A Sesquicentennial History.* Colorado Springs, The Historical Society of the Pikes Peak Region, 1956.

Catlin, George. *Letters and Notes of the Manners, Customs, and Conditions of the North American Indians.* 2 vols. London, privately printed, 1841.

Chandless, William. *A Visit to Salt Lake.* London, Smith, Elder and Co., 1857.

"Charles Denison: [In Memoriam]," *Transactions of the American Climatological Association,* Vol. XXIV (1908), *xxiii.*

Cheever, [Prof.]——. "Colorado as a Sanitarium," *The Peninsular Journal of Medicine* (Detroit), Vol. X (February, 1874), 49–57.

Chicago, Burlington and Quincy Railroad Co. *Eastern Colorado.* Omaha, 1887.

Chittenden, Hiram Martin. *The American Fur Trade of the Far West.* 2 vols. Stanford, Calif., Academic Reprints, 1954.

Chittenden, Newton H. *Health and Pleasure Resorts of the Pacific Coast.* San Francisco, C. A. Murdock and Co., 1884.

Christian, Asa Kyrus. *Mirabeau Buonaparte Lamar.* Austin, Texas, Von Boeckmann–Jones Co., 1922.

The City of San Antonio, Texas. Souvenir Pamphlet, 1902.

Clemens, Samuel L. [Mark Twain, pseud.] *Roughing It.* Hartford, Conn., American Publishing Co., 1884.

Clever, Charles P. *New Mexico: Her Resources; Her Necessities for Railroad Communication with the Atlantic and Pacific States; Her Great Future.* Washington, D.C., McGill and Witherow, 1868.

Clifford, Josephine. "Camp-Life in Arizona," *Overland Monthly,* Vol. IV (March, 1870), 246–52.

Coan, Titus Munson, M.D. "American Mineral Springs," *Chautauquan,* Vol. VII (June, 1887), 543–46.

———. "Climate for Invalids," *Harper's New Monthly Magazine,* Vol. LVIII (March, 1879), 583–89.

Colorado State Board of Health. *Circular No. 9: Consumption and How to Prevent Its Spread in Colorado.* Denver, 1894.

Colorado Territorial Board of Immigration. *Resources and Advantages of Colorado.* Denver, 1873.

Conklin, Enoch. *Picturesque Arizona: Being the Result of Travels and Observations in Arizona During the Fall and Winter of 1877*. New York, The Mining Record Printing Establishment, 1878.

"The Constitution and By-Laws of the American Climatological Association," *Transactions of the American Climatological Association*, Vol. I (1884), 89–94.

"Consumptives Unwelcome in Texas," *Journal of the American Medical Association*, Vol. LII (April 3, 1909), 1118.

"The Cost of Health-seeking," *Scientific American*, Vol. CXII (January 23, 1915), 78.

Cox, Ross. *The Columbia River*. Ed. by Edgar I. and Jane R. Stewart. Norman, University of Oklahoma Press, 1957.

Craig, Robert W., M.D. "Climatography of Arizona, with Especial Reference to the Climatic Treatment of Pulmonary Tuberculosis," *Journal of the American Medical Association*, Vol. XXXVIII (January 25, 1902), 229–33.

———. "Open-Air Treatment of Tuberculosis: Tent Life in Arizona," *Journal of the American Medical Association*, Vol. XXXIX (October 4, 1902), 840–42.

Crimmins, Martin L. "Elliot Roosevelt's Visit to Texas in 1876–1877," *Southwestern Historical Quarterly*, Vol. XLVIII (October, 1944), 186–92.

Crocchiola, Stanley Francis Louis [F. Stanley, pseud.]. *The Las Vegas Story (New Mexico)*. Denver, The World Press, 1951.

———. *Socorro: The Oasis*. Denver, privately printed, 1950.

Crofutt, George A. *Crofutt's Grip-Sack Guide of Colorado: A Complete Encyclopedia of the State, etc.* Omaha, Neb., The Overland Publishing Co., 1881.

Cuming, Fortescue. *Sketches of a Tour to the Western Country, etc.* Vol. IV of Thwaites' *Early Western Travels, q.v.*

Dale, Harrison Clifford, ed. *The Ashley-Smith Explorations and the Discovery of a Central Route to the Pacific 1822–1829*. Glendale, The Arthur H. Clark Co., 1941.

Darlington, Thomas, M.D. "The Doubtful Efficacy of a Hot, Dry Climate in Disease," *Transactions of the American Climatological Association,* Vol. VIII (1891), 234–37.

Davis, Meredith. "Love, Faith and Life: The Story of the Invalid Who Was the Founder of Denver's Craig Colony," *Sunset,* Vol. XLIV (April, 1920), 62–66.

Davis, W. W. H. *El Gringo: New Mexico and Her People.* New York, Harper and Brothers, 1857.

De Cordova, Jacob. *Texas; Her Resources and Her Public Men.* Philadelphia, E. Crozet, 1858.

Delano, Alonzo. *Life on the Plains and Among the Diggings.* Auburn and Buffalo, Miller, Orton and Mulligan, 1854.

Deming, Charles. "Changes in Summer Migration," *The Nation,* Vol. LIII (September 17, 1891), 210–11.

Denison, Charles, M.D. *The Best Welfare of Invalids Seeking the Benefits of Climate: with Suggestions for the Co-operation of Physicians, Life Insurance Officials, etc.* Denver, privately printed, 1875.

———. "The Mineral Springs of Colorado," *Transactions of the American Climatological Association,* Vol. VI (1889), 212–45.

———. "Report on the Climate of Colorado, and Its Relation to Pulmonary Diseases," *Transactions of the American Medical Association,* Vol. XXVII (1876), 456–73.

———. *Rocky Mountain Health Resorts: An Analytical Study of High Altitudes in Relation to the Arrest of Chronic Pulmonary Disease.* Boston, Houghton, Osgood and Co., 1880.

———. "The Sleeping Canopy," *Transactions of the American Climatological Association,* Vol. XXIII (1907), 183–99.

Denver and Rio Grande Railway. *Health, Wealth and Pleasure in Colorado and New Mexico.* Chicago, Belford, Clarke and Co., 1881.

Dickens, Charles. *American Notes.* Boston, Dana Estes and Co., 1868.

Domenech, Emmanuel H. D. *Seven Years' Residence in the Great Deserts of North America.* 2 vols. London, Longman, Green, Longman, and Roberts, 1860.

Dondore, Dorothy Anne. *The Prairie and the Making of Middle America.* Cedar Rapids, Iowa, The Torch Press, 1926.

Drake, Daniel, M.D. *Discourse on the History, Character, and Prospects of the West.* Facsimile reproduction with an introduction by Perry Miller. Gainesville, Fla., Scholars' Facsimiles and Reprints, 1955.

———. *Pioneer Life in Kentucky: A Series of Reminiscential Letters.* Cincinnati, Robert Clarke and Co., 1870.

———. *A Systematic Treatise, Historical, Etiological, and Practical, on the Principal Diseases of the Interior Valley of North America.* Cincinnati, Winthrop B. Smith and Co., 1850.

Dresel, Gustav. *Gustav Dresel's Houston Journal: Adventures in North America and Texas, 1837–1841* Trans. by Max Freund. Austin, University of Texas Press, 1954.

Duffy, John, ed. *The Rudolph Matas History of Medicine in Louisiana.* 2 vols. Baton Rouge, Louisiana State University Press, 1958, 1962.

Durand, Herbert, ed. *San Antonio, Texas: The City of Missions.* St. Louis, Woodward & Tiernan Printing Co., 1894.

Edwards, William A., M.D. "Littoral California," *Transactions of the American Climatological Association,* Vol. XVIII (1902), 122–38.

———, and Beatrice Harraden. *Two-Health-Seekers in Southern California.* Philadelphia, J. B. Lippincott, 1897.

Ehrich, Louis R. *Health Resorts for Lung Troubles.* Colorado Springs, Gazette Publishing Co., 1887.

Eichemeyer, Rudolf. *Letters from the South-West.* New York, J. J. Little and Co., 1894.

El Paso, Texas: A Story of Sunshine. El Paso, El Paso County Medical Society, 1905.

Elliott, Edward E., M.D. "A Practical View of Tent Life in the Southwest," *New York Medical Journal,* Vol. LXXXIV (October 6, 1906), 685–89.

———. "Tenting for Health in the Desert: A Health-Seeker's Advice to Health-Seekers," *The World To-Day,* Vol. XII (April, 1907), 404–13.

Ellis, Amanda M. *Bonanza Towns: Leadville and Cripple Creek.* Spokane, Wash., privately printed, 1954.

Ellison, Edith Nicholl. *The Desert and the Rose.* Boston, The Cornhill Co., 1921.

Emory, William Hemsley. *Lieutenant Emory Reports: A Reprint of Lieutenant W. H. Emory's Notes of a Military Reconnoissance.* Ed. by Ross Calvin. Albuquerque, University of New Mexico Press, 1951.

Engerand, Fernand. "How Our Ancestors Spent Their Holidays," *Review of Reviews* (New York), Vol. IX (January, 1894), 85–86.

Evans, Estwick. *A Pedestrious Tour, of Four Thousand Miles Through the Western States and Territories, etc.* Vol. VIII of Thwaites' *Early Western Travels, q.v.*

Everett, Donald E. "San Antonio Welcomes the 'Sunset'—1877," *Southwestern Historical Quarterly,* Vol. LXV (July, 1961), 49–60.

Farnham, Thomas J. *Travels in the Great Western Prairies, etc.* Vol. XXVIII of Thwaites' *Early Western Travels, q.v.*

Farrand, Livingston. "The First Annual Meeting of the National Association for the Study and Prevention of Tuberculosis, Washington, D.C., May 18 and 19, 1905," *Charities Review,* Vol. XIV (June 3, 1905), 801–806.

Faux, William "Memorable Days in America, etc." In Lindley's *Indiana as Seen by Early Travelers, q.v.*

Field, Matthew C. *Matt Field on the Santa Fe Trail.* Ed. by John E. Sunder. Norman, University of Oklahoma Press, 1960.

———. *Prairie and Mountain Sketches by Matthew C. Field.* Ed. by Kate L. Gregg and John Francis McDermott. Norman, University of Oklahoma Press, 1957.

Fisk, Samuel A., M.D. "Climate in the Cure of Consumption," *Kansas City Review of Science,* Vol. VII (1884), 424–29.

———. "Colorado as a Winter Sanitarium," *Popular Science Monthly,* Vol. XXVIII (March, 1886), 668–79.

———. "Colorado for Invalids," *Popular Science Monthly,* Vol. XXV (July, 1884), 313–20.

———. "Further Considerations of the Analysis of Recorded Cases of Phthisis Pulmonalis," *Transactions of the American Climatological Association,* Vol. VIII (1891), 71–76.

———. "A Search for a Suitable Climate," *Transactions of the American Climatological Association,* Vol. XXIII (1907), 40–52; Vol. XXIV (1908), 15–19.

———. "Some Observations on Southern California," *Transactions of the American Climatological Association,* Vol. XVII (1901), 78–84.

Fitch, William Edward, M.D. *Mineral Waters of the United States and American Spas.* Philadelphia, Lea and Febiger, 1927.

Fitzpatrick, George, ed. *This is New Mexico.* Santa Fe, Bureau of Publications, State of New Mexico, 1948.

Flagg, Edmund. *The Far West: or, a Tour Beyond the Mountains, etc.* Vols. XXVI and XXVII of Thwaites' *Early Western Travels, q.v.*

Flint, Austin, M.D. *A Treatise on the Principles and Practice of Medicine.* 3d ed. Philadelphia, Henry C. Lea, 1868.

Flint, James. *Letters from America, etc.* Vol. IX of Thwaites' *Early Western Travels, q.v.*

Flint, Timothy. *The History and Geography of the Mississippi Valley.* 2d ed. 2 vols in 1. Cincinnati, E. H. Flint and L. R. Lincoln, 1832.

Flower, Richard. *Letters from Lexington and the Illinois, etc.* Vol. X of Thwaites' *Early Western Travels, q. v.*

Forster, William. "Memoirs of William Forster." In Lindley's *Indiana as Seen by Early Travelers, q.v.*

Foscue, Edwin J., and Louis O. Quam. *Estes Park: Resort in the Rockies.* Dallas, The University Press, 1949.

Fossett, Frank. *Colorado: A Historical, Descriptive and Statistical Work on the Rocky Mountain Gold and Silver Mining Region.* Denver, Daily Tribune Steam Printing House, 1876.

———. *Colorado: Its Gold and Silver Mines, Farms and Stock Ranges, and Health and Pleasure Resorts.* New York, C. G. Crawford, 1879.

Fowler, Jacob, *The Journal of Jacob Fowler . . . 1821–22.* Ed. by Elliot Coues. New York, Francis P. Harper, 1898.

Frémont, John C. *Report of the Exploring Expedition to the Rocky Mountains in the Year 1842, and to Oregon and North California in the Years 1843–44.* 28 Cong., 2 sess., *Sen. Exec. Doc. 174.*

Frost, Max, and Paul A. F. Walter, eds. *The Land of Sunshine: A Handbook of the Resources, Industries and Climate of New Mexico.* Santa Fe, New Mexico Board of Managers of the Louisiana Purchase Exposition, 1904.

———. *The Land of Sunshine: A Handbook of the Resources, Products, Industries and Climate of New Mexico.* 2d ed. Santa Fe, New Mexico Territorial Bureau of Immigration, 1906.

Fynn, Arthur J. "Furs and Forts of the Rocky Mountain West," *The Colorado Magazine,* Vol. IX (1932), 45–57, 209–22.

Gallagher, Francis W., M.D. "The Climate of New Mexico," *New York Medical Record,* Vol. XLIX (June 13, 1896), 847–48.

———. "The Rocky Mountain Region, Especially New Mexico," *New York Medical Record,* Vol. XLV (March 10, 1894), 300–301.

Galveston, Harrisburg and San Antonio Railway. *Western Texas as a Winter Resort: via the "Sunset Route."* Chicago, Rand McNally and Co., 1878.

Galveston *News*. January 17, 1871; August 21, 1872.

Gardiner, Charles Fox, M.D. *Doctor at Timberline.* Caldwell, Idaho, The Caxton Printers, Ltd., 1940.

———. "Light and Air in the Treatment of Consumption in Colorado," *Transactions of the American Climatological Association,* Vol. XV (1899), 19–29.

———, "The Sanatory Tent and Its Use in the Treatment of Pulmonary Tuberculosis," *Transactions of the American Climatological Association,* Vol. XVIII (1902), 209–21.

Garrison, Mrs. Gulnare. "Southwestern Texas as a Health Resort," *Medical and Surgical Reporter* (Philadelphia), Vol. XLIV (January 22, 1881), 91–92.

Gatchell, H. P., M. D. *The Invalid's Guide: Where to Go in Search of Health.* Atlanta, James P. Harrison and Co., 1880.

Gerhard, William Wood, M.D. *Lectures on the Diagnosis, Pathology, and Treatment of Diseases of the Chest.* Philadelphia, Haswell and Barrington, 1842.

Gerould, Katharine Fullerton. *The Aristocratic West.* New York, Harper and Brothers, 1925.

Glen, Janet Brownell. "Prisoners of Hope," *The Outlook,* Vol. LVII (October 23, 1897), 474–77.

Godkin, E. L. "Summer Hotels," *The Nation,* Vol. XLI (September 11, 1884), 217–18.

Greatorex, Eliza. *Summer Etchings in Colorado.* New York, G. P. Putnam's Sons, 1873.

Greeley, Horace. *An Overland Journey, from New York to San Francisco in the Summer of 1859.* New York, C. M. Saxton, Barker and Co., 1860.

Green, Rena Maverick, ed. *Samuel Maverick, Texan: 1803–1870.* San Antonio, privately printed, 1952.

Greene, Edward Lee. "Rambles of a Botanist in New Mexico," *American Naturalist*, Vol. XII (March, 1878), 172–76.

Gregg, Josiah. *Commerce of the Prairies*. Ed. by Max L. Moorhead. Norman, University of Oklahoma Press, 1954.

———. *The Commerce of the Prairies*. Ed. by Milo Milton Quaife. Chicago, R. R. Donnelley and Sons, 1926.

———. *Diary and Letters of Josiah Gregg*. Ed. by Maurice Garland Fulton. 2 vols. Norman, University of Oklahoma Press, 1941, 1944.

Hafen, LeRoy R. "Colorado Mountain Men," *The Colorado Magazine*, Vol. XXX (January, 1953), 14–28.

———. "Mountain Men—Andrew W. Sublette," *The Colorado Magazine*, Vol. X (September, 1933), 179–84.

———, and Ann W. Hafen, eds. *To the Rockies and Oregon 1839–1842*. Vol. III of *The Far West and Rockies Historical Series, 1820–1875*. Ed. by LeRoy R. Hafen. 15 vols. Glendale, The Arthur H. Clark Co., 1954–61.

Hale, Albert. "Tuberculosis: Climate and the Great Southwest," *The Reporter Magazine*, Vol. VII (1906), 135–42, 239–46.

Haley, J. Evetts. *Jeff Milton: A Good Man with a Gun*. Norman, University of Oklahoma Press, 1949.

Hall, Sharlot M. "The Burden of the Southwest," *Out West*, Vol. XXVIII (January, 1908), 4–19.

Halley, George, M.D. "New Mexico as a Health Resort," *Kansas City Medical Record*, Vol. V (February, 1888), 41–44.

Hamilton, Patrick. *The Resources of Arizona*. San Francisco, A. L. Bancroft and Co., 1884.

Hamilton, W. T. *My Sixty Years on the Plains*. Ed. by E. T. Sieber. Columbus, Ohio, Long's College Book Co., 1951.

Hardy, Lady Duffus. *Through Cities and Prairie Lands: Sketches of an American Tour*. New York, R. Worthington, 1881.

Harris, Benjamin Butler. *The Gila Trail: The Texas Argonauts and the California Gold Rush.* Ed. by Richard H. Dillon. Norman, University of Oklahoma Press, 1960.

Harris, Dean [William Richard]. *By Path and Trail.* Chicago, Chicago Newspaper Union, 1908.

Hart, James A., M.D. "In Memoriam: Samuel Edwin Solly, M.D., M.R.C.S.," *Transactions of the American Climatological Association,* Vol. XXIII (1907), *xxv–xxvii.*

Hayden, F. V. *The Great West: Its Attractions and Resources.* Philadelphia, Charles R. Brodix, 1880.

Hayes, A. A., Jr., *New Colorado and the Santa Fe Trail.* New York, Harper and Brothers, 1880.

———. "Pioneers of the Sierra Madre," *International Review,* Vol. X (June, 1881), 518–30.

———. "Vacation Aspects of Colorado," *Harper's New Monthly Magazine,* Vol. LX (March, 1880), 542–57.

"Helen Jackson," *The Nation,* Vol. LXI (August 20, 1885), 150–51.

Heustis, Jabez Wiggins. *Physical Observations, and Medical Tracts and Researches, on the Topography and Diseases of Louisiana.* New York, T. and J. Swords, 1817.

Hibbard, William W., M.D. "The Climate of Arizona," *New York Medical Record,* Vol. XLIII (January 28, 1893), 111.

Hill, Emma Shepard. *A Dangerous Crossing and What Happened on the Other Side: Seven Lean Years.* Denver, privately printed, 1924.

Hill, Joseph J. "Antoine Robidoux, Kingpin in the Colorado River Fur Trade, 1824–1844," *The Colorado Magazine,* Vol. VII (July, 1930), 125–31.

Hilzinger, J. George. *Treasure Land: A Story.* Tucson, Arizona Advancement Co., 1897.

Hinsdale, Guy, M.D. "Some Analogous European and American Mineral Springs," *Transactions of the American Climatological Association,* Vol. XVII (1901), 263–65.

Hinton, Richard J. *The Hand-Book to Arizona: Its Resources, History, Towns, Mines, Ruins, and Scenery*. San Francisco, Payot, Upham and Co., 1878. Republished in 1954 by Arizona Silhouettes, Tucson, Arizona.

Hittell, John S. *The Resources of California: Comprising Agriculture, Mining, Geography, Climate, Commerce, etc.* 4th ed. San Francisco and New York, A. Roman and Co., 1868.

Hobby, A. M. "Life of David G. Burnet," *Texas Almanac for 1873*, pp. 158–67. Galveston, W. Richardson and Co., 1872.

Hodge, Frederick Webb, ed. "A Virginian in New Mexico in 1773–74," *New Mexico Historical Review*, Vol. IV (July, 1929), 239–72.

Hodge, Hiram C. *Arizona as It Is: or, The Coming Country, Compiled from Notes of Travel During the Years 1874, 1875, and 1876*. New York, Hurd and Houghton, 1877.

Hoffman, Charles Fenno. *A Winter in the West*. 2 vols. New York, Harper and Brothers, 1835.

Hogan, William Ransom. *The Texas Republic: A Social and Economic History*. Norman, University of Oklahoma Press, 1946.

Holbrook, Stewart H. *The Golden Age of Quackery*. New York, The Macmillan Co., 1959.

Holley, Mary Austin. *Texas [1836]*. A facsimile reprint. Austin, The Steck Company, 1935.

Holme, George. "A Mountain Home for Consumptives," *Munsey's Magazine*, Vol. XXVII (August, 1902), 757–58.

Holmes, Oliver Wendell. *Medical Essays 1842–1882*. Boston, Houghton Mifflin Co., 1888.

Horn, T. G., M.D. "Report on the Mineral Springs of Colorado," *First Annual Report of the Secretary of the State Board of Health, of the State of Colorado* (Denver, 1877), 47–65.

———. "Report on the Mineral Springs of Colorado," *Second*

Annual Report of the State Board of Health of Colorado (Denver, 1878), 43–55.

Hosmer, James K. *A Short History of the Mississippi Valley.* Boston, and New York, Houghton Mifflin Co., 1901.

Houston, Sam. *The Writings of Sam Houston.* Ed. by Amelia W. Williams and Eugene C. Barker. 8 vols. Austin, University of Texas Press, 1938–43.

Howe, Joseph W., M.D. *Winter Homes for Invalids.* New York, G. P. Putnam's Sons, 1875.

Hughes, George W. *Memoir: Descriptive of the March of a Division of the United States Army, under the Command of Brigadier General John E. Wool, from San Antonio de Bexar in Texas, to Saltillo, in Mexico (in 1846).* 31 Cong., 1 sess., *Sen. Exec. Doc. 32.*

Hughes, Thomas, ed. *G. T. T. Gone to Texas.* New York, Macmillan and Co., 1884.

Hulbert, Archer Butler, ed. *Southwest on the Turquoise Trail: The First Diaries on the Road to Santa Fe.* Denver, Stewart Commission of Colorado College and the Denver Public Library, 1933.

Hulme, Thomas. *Journal of a Tour in the Western Countries of America.* Vol. X of Thwaites' *Early Western Travels, q.v.*

Hutchinson, Woods, M.D. "Climate and Health," *The Outing Magazine,* Vol. LIII (March, 1909), 747–53.

———. "Taking the Waters: The Humbug of Hot Springs," *Everybody's Magazine,* Vol. XXVIII (February, 1913), 159–72.

Iddings, Lewis Morris. "Life in the Altitudes: Colorado's Health Plateau," *Scribner's Magazine,* Vol. XIX (February, 1896), 136–51.

Ingersoll, Ernest. *The Crest of the Continent: A Record of a Summer's Ramble in the Rocky Mountains and Beyond.* Chicago, R. R. Donnelley and Sons, 1885.

———. *Knocking Round the Rockies.* New York, Harper and Brothers, 1883.

Irvine, E. Eastman, ed. *The World Almanac and Book of Facts for 1945.* 60th ed. New York, The New York *World-Telegram,* 1945.

Irving, Washington. *Astoria: or Anecdotes of an Enterprise Beyond the Rocky Mountains.* 2 vols. New York and London, G. P. Putnam's Sons, 1895.

Jahns, Pat. *The Frontier World of Doc Holliday.* New York, Hastings House, 1957.

James, Bushrod W., M.D. *American Resorts; with Notes Upon Their Climate.* Philadelphia and London, F. A. Davis, 1889.

James, Edwin. *Account of S. H. Long's Expedition 1819–1820.* Vols. XV to XVII of Thwaites' *Early Western Travels, q.v.*

Jayne, Walter A., M.D. "The Climate of Colorado and Its Effects," *Transactions of the American Climatological Association,* Vol. V (1888), 55–68.

Jebb, Mrs. John G. *A Strange Career: Life and Adventures of John Gladwyn Jebb.* Edinburgh and London, William Blackwood and Sons, 1895.

[Jefferson, Thomas]. *Message from the President of the United States Communicating Discoveries Made in Exploring the Missouri, Red River, and Washita, by Captains Lewis and Clark, Doctor Sibley, and Mr. Dunbar; with a Statistical Account of the Countries Adjacent.* New York, Hopkins and Seymour, 1806.

Johnson, James, M.D. *Change of Air, or the Pursuit of Health; an Autumnal Excursion through France, Switzerland, and Italy, in the Year 1829.* London, S. Highley and T. and G. Underwood, 1831.

Jones, Anson. *Memoranda and Official Correspondence Relating to the Republic of Texas, Its History and Annexation.* New York, D. Appleton and Co., 1859.

Jones Correspondence Files. See explanatory note at the beginning of Bibliography.

Jones, J. J., M.D. "New Mexico as a Health Resort for Consumptives," *Medical and Surgical Reporter* (Philadelphia), Vol. XXXVII (September 15, 1877), 201–203.

Keleher, William A. *The Fabulous Frontier: Twelve New Mexico Items.* Santa Fe, Rydal Press, 1945.

———. *Turmoil in New Mexico, 1846–1868.* Santa Fe, Rydal Press, 1952.

Kellogg, George M., M.D. "New Mexico as a Health Resort," *Journal of the American Medical Association,* Vol. XXVII (September 12, 1896), 582–84.

Kendall, George Wilkins. *Narrative of the Texan Santa Fe Expedition.* Ed. by Milo Milton Quaife. 2 vols in 1. Chicago, The Lakeside Press, 1929.

Kent, C. H. *Texas: The Future Home of the Emigrant.* Davenport, Iowa, Gazette Co., 1878.

Kinder, Francis S. "The Consumptive's Chances in Colorado," *Review of Reviews* (New York), Vol. XXVII (June, 1903), 698–702.

King, Willis P., M.D. *Stories of a Country Doctor.* Philadelphia, Hummel and Parmele, 1891.

Kirkpatrick, John Ervin. *Timothy Flint: Pioneer, Missionary, Author, Editor.* Cleveland, The Arthur H. Clark Co., 1911.

Klebs, Arnold C., M.D. "The Home Treatment of Pulmonary Tuberculosis: Discussion on Home Treatment v. Climatic Treatment of Pulmonary Tuberculosis," *Transactions of the American Climatological Association,* Vol. XVII (1901), 206–13.

Knight, Frederick I., M.D. "The Opening Address," *Transactions of the American Climatological Association,* Vol. I (1884), 2–5.

Knopf, S. A., M.D. "The California Quarantine against Consumptives," *Forum,* Vol. XXVIII (January, 1900), 615–20.

———, "The Tuberculosis Problem in the United States," *North American Review,* Vol. CXLVIII (February, 1899), 212–22.

Knox, R. W., M.D. "Texas Climate in the Trans-Pecos Region," *New York Medical Record,* Vol. LV (April 1, 1899), 461–64.

Krueger, Max. *Pioneer Life in Texas: An Autobiography.* San Antonio, privately printed, 1925.

Langford, J. O., and Fred Gipson. *Big Bend: A Homesteader's Story.* Austin, University of Texas Press, 1952.

Langworthy, Franklin. *Scenery of the Plains, Mountains and Mines: Or a Diary Kept Upon the Overland Route to California, by Way of the Great Salt Lake.* Ogdensburgh, J. C. Sprague, 1855.

Lanier, Sidney. *Retrospects and Prospects: Descriptive and Historical Essays.* New York, Charles Scribner's Sons, 1899.

Larpenteur, Charles. *Forty Years a Fur Trader on the Upper Missouri: The Personal Narrative of Charles Larpenteur 1833–1872.* Ed. by Elliot Coues. 2 vols. New York, Francis P. Harper, 1898.

Las Vegas Hot Springs. 2d ed. Springfield, Ohio, Globe Printing and Publishing Co., 1883.

Las Vegas Southwestern Chautauqua. N.p., n.d.

Latrobe, Benjamin Henry Boneval. *Impressions Respecting New Orleans 1818–1820.* New York, Columbia University Press, 1951.

Lawrence, A. B. *Texas in 1840: Emigrant's Guide to the New Republic.* New York, William W. Allen, 1840.

Lemen, H. A., M.D. "The Influence of the Climate of Colorado on Asthma," *First Annual Report* of the State Board of Health of the State of Colorado (Denver, 1877), 69–73.

Liggett, George S., M.D. "Arizona: A Winter Climate for Consumptives," *New York Medical Journal,* Vol. LIII (March 28, 1891), 367.

Lindley, Harlow, ed. *Indiana as Seen by Early Travelers: A Col-*

lection of Reprints from Books of Travel, Letters, and Diaries Prior to 1830. Indianapolis, Indiana Historical Commission, 1916.

Littlejohn, Eugene M., M.D. "San Antonio and Southwest Texas as a Winter Resort," *New York Medical Record,* Vol. XLII (November 19, 1892), 588.

Lockwood, Frank C. *Arizona Characters.* Los Angeles, Times-Mirror Press, 1928.

Loomis, Alfred L., M.D. "Presidential Address," *Transactions of the American Climatological Association,* Vol. II (1885), 1–14.

Loomis, Noel M. *The Texan–Santa Fe Pioneers.* Norman, University of Oklahoma Press, 1958.

Lowrie, Samuel Harman. *Culture Conflict in Texas 1821–1835.* New York, Columbia University Press, 1932.

McClure, W. K. "Boycott of Consumptives," *The Living Age,* Vol. CCLI (December 8, 1906), 624–29.

McDaniel, H. F., and N. A. Taylor. *The Coming Empire: or, Two Thousand Miles in Texas on Horseback.* New York, A. S. Barnes and Co., 1877.

McGahan, C. F., M.D. "The Climate of the South and Southwest," *Transactions of the American Climatological Association,* Vol. XXV (1909), 98–120.

MacKay, Alex. *The Western World: Travels in the U. S. in 1846–47.* London, Richard Bentley, 1849.

McKay, Seth Shepard. "John Nance Garner," West Texas Historical Association *Year Book,* Vol. XXXVII (October, 1961), 3–44.

McKenna, James A. *Black Range Tales: Chronicling Sixty Years of Life and Adventure in the Southwest.* New York, Wilson-Erickson, Inc., 1936.

McPhail, B. G., M.D. "Special Report on Climatic Influence and Health Resorts of the Western Territories," *Transactions of the Medical Society of Virginia,* Vol. II (1879), 395–401.

Magoffin, Susan Shelby. *Down the Santa Fe Trail: The Diary of Susan Shelby Magoffin, 1846–1847*. Ed. by Stella M. Drumm. New Haven, Yale University Press, 1926.

Mahood, Ruth I. *Photographer of the Southwest.* Los Angeles, The Ward Richie Press, 1961.

Maillard, N. Doran. *The History of the Republic of Texas.* London, Smith, Elder and Co., 1842.

Malone, Dumas, ed. *Dictionary of American Biography.* 20 vols. New York, Charles Scribner's Sons, 1928–36.

Manhattan Medicine Company v. *Wood and Another.* 108 U.S. 218 (1882). Boston, New York, and Washington, Government Printing Office, 1882.

Marchant, Mrs. Mary Jaques. *Texan Ranch Life: with Three Months Through Mexico in a "Prairie Schooner."* London, Horace Cox, 1894.

Mark Twain. See Samuel L. Clemens.

Martin, Edgar W. *The Standard of Living in 1860: American Consumption Levels on the Eve of the Civil War.* Chicago, University of Chicago Press, 1942.

Martineau, Harriet. *Retrospect of Western Travel.* 2 vols. New York, Harper and Brothers, 1838.

———. *Society in America.* New York, Saunders and Otley, 1837.

Masten, H. B., M.D. "New Mexico as a Health Resort," *New York Medical Journal,* Vol. LXXVII (September 6, 1902), 414–17.

Memorial Services Held in the House of Representatives of the United States, Together with Remarks Presented in Eulogy of Bronson Cutting, Late Senator From New Mexico. 74 Cong., 1 sess., *House Doc. 233.*

Miners' Hand-Book and Guide to Pike's Peak. St. Louis, Parker and Huylett, 1859.

Monnette, John W. *History of the Discovery and Settlement of the Valley of the Mississippi.* 2 vols. New York, Harper and Brothers, 1846.

Montule, Edouard de. *Travels in America, 1816–17.* Trans. by Edward D. Seeber. Bloomington, Indiana University Press, 1951.

Moore, B. S., M.D. "The Experience of Syracuse, N.Y., with the Compulsory Tuberculin Test of All Dairies Furnishing Milk to the City," *Journal of the American Medical Association,* Vol. XXXVIII (January 25, 1902), 226–29.

Morrell, Z. N. *Flowers and Fruits in the Wilderness; or Forty-Six Years in Texas and Two Winters in Honduras.* St. Louis, Commercial Printing Co., 1882.

Morris, Maurice O'Connor. *Rambles in the Rocky Mountains: With a Visit to the Gold Fields of Colorado.* London, Smith, Elder and Co., 1864.

"Mrs. Helen Jackson ('H. H.')," *The Century Magazine,* Vol. XXXI (December, 1885), 252–59.

Muir, Andrew Forest, ed. *Texas in 1837: an Anonymous Contemporary Narrative.* Austin, University of Texas Press, 1958.

Mumey, Nolie. *History of the Early Settlements of Denver.* Glendale, The Arthur H. Clark Co., 1942.

Munn, William P. "A Tuberculosis Quarantine Not Practical," *Forum,* Vol. XXIX (April, 1900), 183–87.

Murray, Charles Augustus. *Travels in North America during the Years 1834, 1835, and 1836.* 2 vols. London, Richard Bentley, 1839.

Myers, John Myers. *Doc Holliday.* Boston, Little, Brown and Co., 1955.

National Tuberculosis Association. *A Directory of Sanatoria, Hospitals, Day Camps, and Preventoria for the Treatment of Tuberculosis in the United States.* New York, The Livingston Press, 1931.

New Mexico Territorial Bureau of Immigration. *Bulletin No. 1. New Mexico, 1898: Climate, Mineral Springs, Schools.* Santa Fe, 1898.

Newell, Rev. Chester. *A History of the Revolution in Texas.* A facsimile reprint. Austin, The Steck Co., 1935.

Newman, Oliver P. "Government Care of Consumptives," *Review of Reviews* (New York), Vol. XXX (July, 1904), 59–64.

Nicholl, Edith M. *Observations of a Ranchwoman in New Mexico.* London, Macmillan and Co., Ltd., 1898.

Nichols, C. F., M.D. "The Service of an Invalid Aid Society," *Review of Reviews* (New York), Vol. XI (March, 1895), 290–92.

Nichols, Thomas Low, M.D. *Forty Years of American Life, 1821–1861.* New York, Stackpole Sons, 1937.

Nixon, Pat Ireland, M.D. *A Century of Medicine in San Antonio.* Lancaster, Pa., Lancaster Press, 1936.

Nordhoff, Charles. *California: for Health, Pleasure, and Residence.* New York, Harper and Brothers, 1873.

North, Thomas. *Five Years in Texas.* Cincinnati, Street Printing Co., 1870.

Nuttall, Thomas. *A Journal of Travels into the Arkansas Territory, etc.* Vol. XIII of Thwaites' *Early Western Travels, q.v.*

"Obituary: Dr. Jeremiah T. Eskridge," *Transactions of the American Climatological Association,* Vol. XVIII (1902), *xxxi–xxxii.*

Oliver, William. *Eight Months in Illinois: With Advice to Immigrants.* Chicago, Walter M. Hill, 1924. Reprint of 1843 edition.

Olmsted, Frederick Law. *A Journey Through Texas: A Saddle Trip on the Southwestern Frontier.* New York, Mason Bros., 1860.

Opportunities for the Homeseeker: Texas, the Coming Country, the Newest Southwest. San Antonio, Hust and Brundage, [1905?].

Orme, H. S., M.D. "Climate of Southern California," *Transactions of the American Climatological Association,* Vol. IV (1887), 143–55.

Otis, Edward O., M.D. "Some Observations on Health Resorts," *Journal of the American Medical Association,* Vol. VI (March 20, 1886), 316–19.

Palmer, E. Payne, M.D. "Phoenix, Arizona, as a Health Resort for Tuberculous Patients," *New York Medical Journal,* Vol. LXXII (November 17, 1900), 852–54.

Palmer, William J. *Report of the Surveys Across the Continent in 1867–68 on the Thirty-fifth and Thirty-second Parallels.* Philadelphia, W. B. Selkeimer, 1869.

Parker, Amos Andrew. *Trip to the West and Texas.* Concord, N.H., White and Fisher, 1835.

Parker, Rev. Samuel. *Journal of an Exploring Tour Beyond the Rocky Mountains in the Years 1835, '36, and '37.* 3d ed. Ithaca, N.Y., Mack, Andrus, and Woodruff, 1842.

Parker, William Thornton, M.D. "Shall We Have a National Sanitarium for Consumptives?" *The Arena,* Vol. XVI (July, 1896), 196–206.

Parrish, Edward Evans. *Crossing the Plains in 1844.* N.p., 1844.

"Patent Medicine Suits," *The Medical and Surgical Reporter* (Philadelphia), Vol. LI (July 26, 1884), 101–102.

Peale, Albert C., M.D. "The Classification of American Mineral Waters," *Transactions of the American Climatological Association,* Vol. IV (1887), 156–66.

Peplow, Edward H., Jr. *History of Arizona.* 2 vols. New York, Lewis Historical Publishing Company, Inc., 1958.

Perrigo, Lynn I. *Historical Sites in and near the "Meadow City."* Las Vegas, N.M., The Las Vegas–San Miguel Chamber of Commerce, 1963.

Perrin du Lac, François Marie. *Travel Through the Two Loui-*

sianas and Among the Savage Nations of the Missouri; In the United States, Along the Ohio, and the Adjacent Provinces. London, Richard Phillips by J. G. Barnard, 1807.

Pickard, Madge E., and R. Carlyle Buley. *The Midwest Pioneer: His Ills, Cures, and Doctors.* New York, Henry Schuman, 1946.

Pike, Zebulon Montgomery. *The Expeditions of Zebulon Montgomery Pike, to the Headwaters of the Mississippi River, Through Louisiana Territory, and in New Spain, During the Years 1805–6–7.* Ed. by Elliot Coues. 2 vols. London and New York, Simpkin, Marshall, Hamilton, Kent and Co., Ltd., and Francis P. Harper, 1895.

Pine, George W. *Beyond the West.* Utica, N.Y., T. J. Griffiths, 1870.

Pomeroy, Earl. *In Search of the Golden West: The Tourist in Western America.* New York, Alfred A. Knopf, 1957.

Powers, Stephen. *Afoot and Alone: A Walk from Sea to Sea.* Hartford, Conn., Columbian Book Co., 1872.

———. "Solid Days in Texas," *Overland Monthly,* Vol. VI (June, 1871), 555–61.

"The Problem of Poor Lungers Who Go West," *The Survey,* Vol. XXXII (April 18, 1914), 67.

"Professional Quacks," *The Medical and Surgical Reporter* (Philadelphia), Vol. LI (December 13, 1884), 697.

"Quack Medicine Advertisements," *The Medical and Surgical Reporter* (Philadelphia), Vol. LI (November 29, 1884), 627–28.

Quaife, Milo Milton, ed. *Pictures of Gold Rush California.* Chicago, R. R. Donnelley and Sons, 1949.

Rae, W. F. *Westward by Rail: The New Route to the East.* New York, D. Appleton and Company, 1871.

Ralph, Julian. "Colorado's Unique Resort," *Harper's Weekly Magazine,* Vol. XXXVIII (March 17, 1894), 253.

———. *Our Great West: A Study of the Present Conditions and*

Future Possibilities of the New Commonwealths and Capitals of the United States. New York, Harper and Brothers, 1893.

Rawlings, Isaac D. *The Rise and Fall of Disease in Illinois.* 2 vols. Springfield, Ill., State Department of Public Health, 1927.

Reed, Isaac. "The Christian Traveler, 1828." In Lindley's *Indiana as Seen by Early Travelers, q.v.*

Reeve, Frank D. *History of New Mexico.* 2 vols. New York, Lewis Historical Publishing Co., Inc., 1961.

Regan, John. *The Emigrant's Guide to the Western States of America: or Backwoods and Prairies.* Edinburgh, Oliver and Boyd, 1852.

Reynolds, John. *Reynolds' History of Illinois: My Own Times, Also the History of My Life.* Chicago, Fergus Printing Co., 1879.

Richards, George L., M.D. *Consumption: Cases that Should Go to Colorado and Cases that Should Remain at Home.* Fall River, Mass., privately printed, 1898.

Richardson, Albert D. *Beyond the Mississippi: From the Great River to the Great Ocean.* Hartford, Conn., American Publishing Co., 1867.

———. *Our New States and Territories, Being Notes of a Recent Tour of Observation through Colorado, Utah, Idaho, Nevada, Oregon, Montana, Washington Territory and California.* New York, Beadle and Company, 1866.

Ritch, William G. *New Mexico, Historical and Industrial.* 5th ed. Santa Fe, Territorial Bureau of Immigration, 1885.

Rock, James L. and W. I. Smith. *Southern and Western Texas Guide.* St. Louis, A. H. Granger, 1878.

Rockwell, William S. *Colorado: Its Mineral and Agricultural Resources.* New York, privately printed, 1864.

Rodgers, Mark A., M.D. "The Climate of Arizona," *Transactions of the American Climatological Association,* Vol. XII (1896), 88–105.

———. "Some Observations on Tuberculosis by a Dweller in the Desert," *Charities Review,* Vol. XVI (September 1, 1906), 558–63.

Rosenboom, Eugene H., and Francis P. Weisenburger. *A History of Ohio.* Columbus, Ohio State Archaeological and Historical Society, 1958.

Ruedi, Carl, M.D. "A Comparison of the Winter Health-Resorts in the Alps with Some Places in the Rocky Mountains of Colorado," *Transactions of the American Climatological Association,* Vol. X (1893–94), 28–42.

Rush, Benjamin, M.D. *An Inquiry into the Various Sources of the Usual Forms of Summer and Autumnal Disease in the United States.* Philadelphia, J. Conrad and Co., 1805.

———. *Observations Upon the Origin of the Malignant Bilious, or Yellow Fever in Philadelphia, and Upon the Means of Preventing It.* Philadelphia, Thomas Dobson, 1799.

Russell, William L., M.D. "Consumption and Consumptives," *Popular Science Monthly,* Vol. L (January, 1897), 336–44.

Ruxton, George Frederick. *Ruxton of the Rockies.* Ed. by LeRoy R. Hafen. Norman, University of Oklahoma Press, 1950.

Ryus, W. H. *The Second William Penn: A True Account of Incidents that Happened Along the Old Santa Fe Trail in the Sixties.* Kansas City, Mo., Frank T. Tiley, 1913.

Sage, Rufus B. *Scenes in the Rocky Mountains and in Oregon, California, New Mexico, Texas, and the Grand Prairies.* Philadelphia, Carey and Hart, 1846.

Sajous, Charles E., ed. *Annual of the Universal Sciences.* Philadelphia, F. A. Davis, 1891.

San Miguel County, New Mexico. Santa Fe, New Mexico Bureau of Immigration, 1908.

Sanborn, C. A., M.D. "The Climate of the Eastern Foothills of Southern California," *Transactions of the American Climatological Association,* Vol. XVIII (1902), 92–95.

Schallenberger, Moses. *The Opening of the California Trail: The Story of the Stevens Party as Set Down by H. H. Bancroft.* Ed. by George R. Stewart. Berkeley, University of California Press, 1953.

Schauffler, E. W., M.D. "The Climate of El Paso, Texas," *Transactions of the American Climatological Association,* Vol. III (1886), 209–13.

Schoolcraft, Henry R. *Personal Memoirs of a Residence of Thirty Years with the Indian Tribes.* Philadelphia, Lippincott, Grambo and Co., 1851.

Schroeder, Henry H., M.D. "A Study of Highly Mineralized Thermal Waters in the Treatment of Disease, Based on Experience at the Glenwood Hot Springs, Colorado," *Transactions of the American Climatological Association,* Vol. XII (1896), 225–45.

Scobee, Barry. "History Obscures Tent City," San Angelo (Texas) *Standard-Times,* February 14, 1960.

"The Search for Health," *Spectator,* Vol. LXXXVII (September 21, 1901), 382–83.

"On Sen. Clinton P. Anderson: Anderson to Succeed Kerr as Space Committee Chairman," *Congressional Quarterly Fact Sheet,* January 21, 1963,1–2.

Sewell, Henry, M.D. *Some Considerations on the Climatic Treatment of Consumption with Especial Reference to Denver as a Health Resort.* Chicago, n.p., 1903.

Shryock, Richard Harrison. *Medicine and Society in America, 1660–1860.* New York, New York University Press, 1960.

Sibley, George Champlin. *The Road to Santa Fe: The Journal and Diaries of George Champlin Sibley.* Ed. by Kate L. Gregg. Albuquerque, University of New Mexico Press, 1952.

Silliman, B——. "On Some of the Mining Districts near the Rió Colorado, with Remarks on the Climate, etc.," *The American*

Journal of Science and Arts, [n.s.] Vol. XLI (May, 1866), 289–308.

Sims, J. Marion, M.D. *The Story of My Life.* New York, D. Appleton and Co., 1886.

Smith, Frank. *The Yazoo River.* New York, Rinehart and Co., 1954.

Solly, Samuel Edwin, M.D. "Climatology as a Study in the Medical Schools," *Transactions of the American Climatological Association,* Vol. XX (1904), 7–13.

———. "The Comparative Merits of Resorts in New Mexico, Colorado, and Arizona," *Transactions of the American Climatological Association,* Vol. XIII (1897), 171–85.

———. "An Invalid's Day in Colorado Springs," *Transactions of the American Climatological Association,* Vol. IV (1887), 173–84.

———. "Invalids Suited for Treatment at Colorado Springs," *Transactions of the American Climatological Association,* Vol. V (1888), 23–35.

———. *Manitou, Colorado, U.S.A., Its Mineral Waters and Climate.* St. Louis, John McKittrick and Co., 1875.

———. "Presidential Address: The Principles of Medical Climatology," *Transactions of the American Climatological Association,* Vol. XI (1895), 1–8.

———. "Treatment of Pulmonary Consumption by Residence in Colorado as Exemplified by the Analysis of 141 Cases," *Transactions of the American Climatological Association,* Vol. VII (1890), 132–62.

———, and Mrs. Simeon J. Dunbar. *The Health Resorts of Colorado Springs and Manitou: also A Prize Article, Descriptive of Scenery, Resources, etc.* Colorado Springs, The Gazette Publishing Co., 1883.

Sowell, Andrew Jackson. *Heroes of Texas: Deaf Smith.* Houston, The Union National Bank, 1929.

Sprague, J. R. "Progress and Resources of Texas," *DeBow's Review,* Vol. XXVI (April, 1859), 471–74.

Standard, A. C., M.D. "The Climate of the Great Salt Lake Basin," *Transactions of the American Climatological Association,* Vol. VII (1890), 72–80.

Stanley, F. See Stanley F. L. Crocchiola.

Steele, Edward Dunsha. *Edward Dunsha Steele, 1829–1865: Pioneer, Schoolteacher, Cabinetmaker, and Musician: A Diary of His Journey from Lodi, Wisconsin, Across the Plains to Boulder, Colorado, in the Year 1859.* Ed. by Nolie Mumey. Boulder, Johnson Publishing Co., 1960.

Steele, John. *In Camp and Cabin: Mining Life and Adventure in California During 1850 and Later.* Ed. by Milo Milton Quaife. Chicago, The Lakeside Press, 1928.

Stevens, Walter B. *Through Texas.* St. Louis, n.p., 1890.

———. *Through Texas. A Series of Interesting Letters.* St. Louis, St. Louis Southwestern Railway, 1892. Another edition, 1893.

Stoddard, Amos. *Sketches, Historical and Descriptive, of Louisiana.* Philadelphia, Mathew Carey, 1812.

Stolley, Richard B. "The Senator's [Barry Goldwater's] Pioneer Mother Talks About Barry and Herself," *Life,* Vol. LV (July 12, 1963), 25–26.

Stubbert, J. Edward, M.D. "Tent Life for Consumptives," *Transactions of the American Climatological Association,* Vol. XIX (1903), 88–100.

Sunder, John E. *Bill Sublette, Mountain Man.* Norman, University of Oklahoma Press, 1959.

Sweet, Alexander E., and J. Amory Knox. *On a Mexican Mustang, Through Texas, From the Gulf to the Río Grande.* Hartford, Conn., S. S. Scranton and Co., 1883.

———. *Sketches from "Texas Siftings."* New York, Texas Siftings Publishing Co., 1882.

Taylor, Bayard. *Colorado: A Summer Trip.* New York, G. P. Putnam and Son, 1867.

———. *Eldorado; or Adventures in the Path of Empire.* Introduction by Robert Glass Cleland. New York, Alfred A. Knopf, 1949.

Taylor, Charles Fayette, M.D. "Climate and Health," *Popular Science Monthly,* Vol. XLVII (July, 1895), 313–26.

Taylor, F. H. "Through Texas," *Harper's New Monthly Magazine,* Vol. LIX (October, 1879), 703–18.

Taylor, M. K. "The Climate of Southwestern Texas and Its Advantages as a Winter Health Resort," *Transactions of the American Climatological Association,* Vol. V (1888), 209–20.

Teas, Thomas Scattergood. "Journal of a Tour to Fort Wayne . . . in the Year 1821." In Lindley's *Indiana as Seen by Early Travelers, q.v.*

Teetor, Henry Dudley. "Letter from Manitou Springs," *Magazine of Western History,* Vol. XIII (February, 1891), 435–42.

———. "Manitou Springs, All The Year Round," *Magazine of Western History,* Vol. XI (November, 1889), 43–47.

———. "One Summer Day at Idaho Springs," *Magazine of Western History,* Vol. XIII (November, 1890), 15–19.

———. "A Pioneer of Manitou Springs," *Magazine of Western History,* Vol. XIII (December, 1890), 159–61.

———. "Some of the Mineral Springs of Colorado," *Magazine of Western History,* Vol. XIII (January, 1891), 304–307.

Tenney, Edward P. *Colorado: New Homes in the West.* Boston, Lee and Shepard, 1880.

"Tent Cottages for Consumptives," *Charities Review,* Vol. X (May 9, 1903), 516–17.

Texas Almanac for [*1857–1868*] . . . . Galveston, W. Richardson and Co., 1858–68.

Texas Almanac and Emigrant's Guide to Texas, etc. Galveston, W. Richardson and Co., 1869–72; Galveston, Richardson, Belo and Co., 1873.

Texas Almanac and State Industrial Guide. Dallas, A. H. Belo, 1904, 1910, 1912, 1914.

"Texas' Carlsbad," *The Texas and Pacific Quarterly,* Vol. VIII (July, 1905), 27–31.

Thayer, William M. *Marvels of the New West.* Norwich, Conn., The Henry Bell Publishing Co., 1888.

"Things Wise and Otherwise," *Harper's Weekly Magazine,* January 3, 1857, p. 14; May 2, 1857, p. 286.

Thomas, David. "Travels Through the Western Country in the Summer of 1816." In Lindley's *Indiana as Seen by Early Travelers, q.v.*

Thornton, J. Quinn. *Oregon and California in 1848.* 2 vols. New York, Harper and Brothers, 1849.

Thwaites, Reuben Gold, ed. *Early Western Travels, 1748–1846.* 32 vols. Cleveland, The Arthur H. Clark Co., 1904–1907.

Tice, John T. *Over the Plains and on the Mountains: In Kansas and Colorado.* St. Louis, Industrial Age Printing Co., 1872.

Timmons, Bascom N. *Garner of Texas: A Personal History.* New York, Harper and Brothers, 1948.

Tinkle, Lon, and Allen Maxwell, eds. *The Cowboy Reader.* New York, London, and Toronto, Longmans, Green and Co., 1959.

Triplett, Frank. *Conquering the Wilderness; or, a New Pictorial History of the Life and Times of the Pioneer Heroes and Heroines of America.* New York and London, N. D. Thompson and Co., 1883.

Trollope, Frances (Milton). *Domestic Manners of the Americans.* 2 vols. London, Whittaker, Treacher and Co., 1832.

Turner, Thomas. "Eager Empire," *Texas Parade,* Vol. XX (April, 1960), 28–31.

———. "Early Health Resort Lives Only in Memory," Dallas *Morning News,* February 17, 1948.

Union Pacific Railway Company. *Colorado: A Complete and Comprehensive Description; the Resources and Attractions of*

Colorado for the Home Seeker and the Tourist. Battle Creek, 1890.

Van Bibber, W. C., M.D. "The Therapeutic Value of Some of the Mineral Waters of the United States upon Malarial Diseases; with Rules for their Use," *Transactions of the American Climatological Association,* Vol. V (1888), 237–44.

Volney, C. F. "A View of the Soil and Climate of the United States of America (1804)." In Lindley's *Indiana as Seen by Early Travelers, q.v.*

Wagner, Clinton, M.D. "Colorado Springs and Davos-Platz, as Winter Health Resorts, Compared," *New York Medical Record,* Vol. XXXII (October 29, 1887), 567–70.

Walker, James B., M.D. "Presidential Address: Some of the Difficulties of Climato-Therapy," *Transactions of the American Climatological Association,* Vol. XII (1896), 1–12.

———. "Some Remarks on Climate and Renal Diseases," *Transactions of the American Climatological Association,* Vol. XV (1899), 99–107.

Wallace, Susan E. *The Land of the Pueblos.* New York, George D. Hurst, 1888.

Wallian, Samuel Spencer, M.D. "The Search for Health," *Junior Munsey,* Vol. VIII (1900), 463–68.

Warner, Charles Dudley. "The Outlook of Southern California," *Harper's New Monthly Magazine,* Vol. LXXXII (January, 1891), 167–89.

Watkins, W. Warner, M.D. "Ignorance or Malpractice: Financial and Climatic Conditions in the Treatment of Tuberculosis," *Journal of the American Medical Association,* Vol. LII (April 10, 1909), 1175–76.

Waxham, F. E., M. D. "The Outdoor Treatment of Tuberculosis," *Journal of American Medical Association,* Vol. XXXIX (November 29, 1902), 1392–93.

Webb, James Josiah. *Adventures in the Santa Fé Trade 1844–*

1847. Vol. I in Ralph P. Bieber's *The Southwest Historical Series, q.v.*

Webb, Walter Prescott, ed. *The Handbook of Texas*. 2 vols. Austin, The Texas State Historical Association, 1952.

Weber, Hermann, M.D. "Manitou in Colorado (U.S.A.): A Health Resort in Consumption," *The Lancet* (London), Vol. II (August 4, 1877), 156–58.

Welby, Adlard. *A Visit to North America and the English Settlements in Illinois, etc.* Vol. XII of Thwaites' *Early Western Travels, q.v.*

Wetherill, H. G., M.D. "Health-Resorts of the West and Southwest," *Medical News* (Philadelphia), Vol. LXIII (December 16, 1893), 681–83.

Wharton, Clarence R., ed. *Texas Under Many Flags*. 5 vols. Chicago and New York, The American Historical Society, Inc., 1930.

Wheeler, A. C. "On the Iron Trail," *Scribner's Magazine*, Vol. XII (August, 1876), 529–43.

Williams, Joseph. *The Joseph Williams Tour*. Vol. III in LeRoy R. and Ann W. Hafen, eds., *The Far West and Rockies Historical Series, 1820–1875, q.v.*

Williams, O. W. "From Dallas to the Site of Lubbock in 1877," West Texas Historical Association *Year Book*, Vol. XV (1939), 3–21.

Wilson, Alexander M. "A Summer Camp for Tuberculosis," *Charities Review*, Vol. XIV (September 2, 1905), 1045–46.

Wilson, John. *Health and Health Resorts*. Philadelphia, Porter and Coates, 1880.

Wilson, William E. *The Wabash*. New York, Farrar and Rinehart, 1940.

Wingate, U. O. B. "National Health Legislation," *North American Review*, Vol. CXLVII (November, 1898), 527–33.

Winslow, Charles-Edward Amory. *The Conquest of Epidemic*

Disease: A Chapter in the History of Ideas. Princeton, Princeton University Press, 1944.

Wislizenus, Frederick Adolphus. *Memoir of a Tour to Northern Mexico, Connected with Col. Doniphan's Expedition, in 1846 and 1847.* 30 Cong., 1 sess., *Sen. Misc. Doc. 26.*

Woods, John. *Two Years' Residence . . . in the Illinois Country, United States.* Vol. X of Thwaites' *Early Western Travels, q.v.*

Worth, James H., M.D. "The Climate of New Mexico as Viewed by the Medical Fraternity There," *Transactions of the American Climatological Association,* Vol. VII (1890–91), 285–90.

Wright, Solomon Alexander. *My Rambles as East Texas Cowboy, Hunter, Fisherman, Tie-Cutter.* Austin, Texas Folklore Society, 1942.

Wyeth, John B. *Oregon: A Short History of a Long Journey, etc.* Vol. XXI of Thwaites' *Early Western Travels, q.v.*

Yandell, W. M., M.D. "The Preferable Attributes of Climate for Consumption, as Applied to the Winters in Southern New Mexico, Southern Arizona, and Western Texas," *Transactions of the American Climatological Association,* Vol. VII (1890), 81–100.

Yard, Robert Sterling. *The National Parks Portfolio.* Washington, D.C., U.S. Government Printing Office, 1921.

Young, James Harvey. "American Medical Quackery in the Age of the Common Man," *Mississippi Valley Historical Review,* Vol. XLVII (March, 1961), 579–93.

Ziegler, Jesse A. *Wave of the Gulf.* San Antonio, The Naylor Company, 1938.

Index

The text for *Health-Seekers in the Southwest, 1817–1900* has been set on the Linotype in 11-point Caledonia, a distinguished type designed by the late W. A. Dwiggins, eminent American graphic artist. The book is printed by letterpress on a paper which bears the watermark of the University of Oklahoma Press, and which has an effective life of at least three hundred years.

University of Oklahoma Press
Norman